How to Assess Doctors and Health Professionals

How to Assess Doctors and Health Professionals

Mike Davis
Consultant in Continuing Medical Education, Blackpool, UK

Judy McKimm
Professor and Dean of Medical Education, Swansea University, Swansea, UK

Kirsty Forrest
Consultant Anaesthetist, Leeds Teaching Hospital Trust, Leeds, UK

with
Steve Capey
Jacky Hanson
Kamran Khan

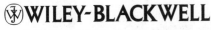
A John Wiley & Sons, Ltd., Publication

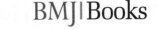

This edition first published 2013, © 2013 by Blackwell Publishing Ltd

Blackwell Publishing was acquired by John Wiley & Sons in February 2007. Blackwell's publishing program has been merged with Wiley's global Scientific, Technical and Medical business to form Wiley-Blackwell.

Registered office: John Wiley & Sons, Ltd, The Atrium, Southern Gate, Chichester, West Sussex, PO19 8SQ, UK

Editorial offices: 9600 Garsington Road, Oxford, OX4 2DQ, UK
The Atrium, Southern Gate, Chichester, West Sussex, PO19 8SQ, UK
111 River Street, Hoboken, NJ 07030-5774, USA

For details of our global editorial offices, for customer services and for information about how to apply for permission to reuse the copyright material in this book please see our website at www.wiley.com/wiley-blackwell.

Library of Congress Cataloging-in-Publication Data

How to assess doctors and health professionals / Mike Davis ... [et al.].
      p. ; cm.
   Includes bibliographical references and index.
   ISBN 978-1-4443-3056-4 (paper)
   I. Davis, Mike, 1947-
   [DNLM: 1. Education, Medical–standards.   2. Educational Measurement–methods.
3. Clinical Competence–standards.   4. Education, Professional–standards.   W 18]
   610.711–dc23
                            2012041073

A catalogue record for this book is available from the British Library.

Wiley also publishes its books in a variety of electronic formats. Some content that appears in print may not be available in electronic books.

Cover design by: Meaden Creative

Set in 9.5/12 pt Minion Regular by Toppan Best-set Premedia Limited
Printed and bound in Malaysia by Vivar Printing Sdn Bhd

1   2013

Contents

Acknowledgements

Judy McKimm and Kirsty Forrest would like to say thank you to students, colleagues, family and friends for their wisdom, insights and support which have helped shape and inform this book.

Mike Davis would like to thank friends and colleagues from ALSG/ RC(UK) Generic Instructor Course communities for their input into his thinking for some time. He would also like to give special thanks to Christine for insight, encouragement and support, particularly over the past 18 months.

Thanks also to Alison Quinn for her contributions to the chapters on assessment types.

About the authors

Lead authors

Mike Davis is a freelance consultant in continuing medical education. He is lead educator with Advanced Life Support Group where he has been involved in the development of the virtual learning environments elements across a wide range of blended courses. He is an educator with the ATLS instructor course, the Royal College of Surgeons' Train the Trainer course, and was lead educator during the development and refinement of the European Trauma Course.

Judy McKimm is Professor and Dean of Medical Education at Swansea University. She has wide experience in undergraduate and postgraduate medical and healthcare education and her research and publications are primarily in medical education, teaching and learning, educational and clinical leadership development and professional practice. She has worked in many countries on educational and health management capacity building initiatives, most recently in the Pacific.

Kirsty Forrest is a consultant anaesthetist in Leeds. She is also clinical education advisor for the Yorkshire and Humber Deanery and co-chair of the Student Selected Components course of the MBChB at Leeds University. She has been involved in educational research for 10 years and awarded funding via a university fellowship and the Higher Education Academy. She is co-author and editor of a number of best-selling medical textbooks.

Additional authors

Steve Capey initially trained as a pharmacologist at the University of Wales College of Medicine and is currently the Assessment Director for the MBBCh programme at the Swansea University College of Medicine. He has been instrumental in the development of new medical curricula at Keele and Swansea. His research interests are in innovative integrated assessment systems and he has presented his findings at national and international conferences on medical education and assessment.

Jacky Hanson is a consultant in emergency medicine at Lancashire Teaching Hospitals NHS Trust (LTHTR). She has taught extensively at undergraduate and postgraduate levels and on Advanced Life Support courses. She is the Director of the Lancashire Simulation Centre, LTHTR involved in training in both clinical and human factor skills, using blended learning. She was Director of Continuing Professional Development and Revalidation for the College of Emergency Medicine. She is an examiner for the Fellowship of the College of Emergency Medicine.

Kamran Khan has developed a passion for medical education and acquired higher qualification in this field alongside his parent speciality in anaesthetics. He has been in clinical academic posts, first at the University of Oxford and currently at the University of Manchester. He is Associate lead for Assessments at the Manchester Medical School. He has extensively presented and published at the national and international levels in his fields of academic interest.

Alison Quinn has taken a year out of an anaesthetic training programme for a Fellowship in Medical Education and Simulation. She also holds an honorary lecturer post with the University of Manchester, Medical School, working in the Assessments Team. She is also studying for a Post Graduate Certificate in Medical Education.

Foreword

Well done for picking up this small tome. Keep reading, you will find its contents important.

First, ask yourself why you should be interested in assessment? After all, it is going to be another drain on your time and may result in first hand experience of conflict resolution with examinees and other examiners.

One reason is something you know from your own personal experience: all tests need to ensure they are fair and up-to-date. Abdicating responsibility increases the chance that they will dumb down to the lowest common denominator. This may achieve a target of some central committee but it is unlikely to help the patient who is being cared for by a medical practitioner with substandard abilities.

Although the medical profession is replete with assessments, they are not a panacea for other educational problems. It is therefore important to understand what they can and cannot do. Properly constructed and used, assessments can provide a powerful, positive educational experience which motivates the learner to move on to higher levels of competence. In contrast, a poorly constructed or applied assessment can produce practitioners with little confidence and highly developed avoidance strategies for the subject.

After many years as examinees, we typically find our initial involvement with assessment may be as instructors on courses or examiners of medical students in formative assessments. Later on, we may become involved with high stakes examinations such as university finals and college diplomas. Subsequently, some of us become part of a team devising and developing assessments. Running alongside this is our own professional need to keep taking further assessments, either as part of a chosen speciality training programme or to complete revalidation. This book provides you with the key information needed to carry out these various roles. The authors have taken a pragmatic approach, covering the educational theory in as much detail as is required to understand the strengths and weaknesses of the various assessment tools that you will come across.

There is no ideal single tool in existence that can adequately assess the range of cognitive, psychomotor and affective competences that are required to practice as a medical student, trainee or specialist. Inevitably, those abilities that are easiest to measure are not necessarily the most important – especially as the training evolves and deeper learning occurs. The authors therefore describe how to use a collection of tests, with each component targeted at specific competencies listed in the curriculum. They also show that having the tests linked to the educational outcome enables the examination and teaching to reinforce one another. When assessment develops as an afterthought, it invariably fails to meet the range and depth required to ensure the appropriate level of skill has been achieved.

The important role assessment has in learning is often forgotten and powerful learning opportunities are missed. The authors address this by discussing the educational potential in both formative and summative assessments. This obviously brings up the issue of feedback and how this can be best carried out. Failing an assessment is never pleasant, particularly when it is a high stakes exam. These examinees will therefore present a range of needs and emotions. In some cases this can result in people resorting to litigation when they feel incorrect decisions have been made. Examiners, and their boards, therefore need to be absolutely sure that the competences assessed were suitable and carried out in an approved way using the optimal tools. In this way appropriate feedback and advice can be given. Furthermore, those involved in the assessment can be confident when questioned, sometimes in a court of law, as to the decisions they made.

The holy grail of any medical educational programme is to produce an improvement in patient care. Consequently, assessments should ideally be carried out in the workplace. This book provides advice on balancing the often conflicting desires of validity, reliability, specificity, feasibility and fidelity. Such a strategy also involves the use of learning technologies as they can help with assessment development, its administration, marking and analysis. e-Portfolios are another manifestation of computer-assisted learning and assessment that examiners need to be familiar with. How learning technologies can be best used, and errors to avoid, are addressed by the authors.

Therefore I hope you continue to read this book as it will make the process of assessment more transparent, relevant and comprehensible. You will then be able to bring these same qualities to the next assessment you carry out.

Peter Driscoll
BSc, MD, FCEM
Honorary Senior Lecturer, School of Medicine,
University of St Andrews
Professor, College of Emergency Medicine

Preface

This book is designed to complement an earlier volume in the *How to . . .* series, *How to Teach Continuing Medical Education* by Mike Davis and Kirsty Forrest, and is intended to fill the very obvious gap in that edition. This is not to suggest, however, that assessment is an afterthought. As Harden wrote:

> *Assessment should be seen as integral to any course or training programme and not merely an add-on* [1].

There is a tendency to take assessment for granted in the early years of a career in medical education and not to question why assessments are structured in the way that they are. Medical education is fairly idiosyncratic in the way that it assesses learners. In addition to more conventional assessments such as essays, multiple choice questions or presentations, assessment methods such as Objective Structured Clinical Examinations (OSCEs), long cases, Extended Matching Questions (EMQs) and Mini Clinical Evaluation Exercises (mini-CEXs) are primarily used only in medical education. Students and trainees on the whole are usually on the receiving end of assessment rather than acting as assessors themselves and, in the same way that fish are not conscious of the water, trainees are submerged in the assessment environment and it only impinges on them when there is some kind of cathartic event, usually associated with not achieving a desired standard.

All of us have been involved in assessment at one time or another. We have certainly all had important decisions made about our careers on the basis of assessments. Many of us have also been involved in the assessment of students or trainees at some point in our career; however, not all of us have considered the evidence base that surrounds assessment. We would not consider making life-changing decisions about a patient without having an understanding of the condition they are suffering from and the same is true about assessment. When we assess students in high stakes exams we are making decisions about them that could have life-changing potential.

What this book is designed to do is make explicit some of the characteristics of different types of assessments from the point of view of assessors
and clinical teachers. It explores some of the theories associated with assessment and examines how these are manifested in what assessors do and why
and in a variety of settings, ranging from the informal to the most formal.
Each chapter includes some activities and considers the issues around the
experiences of the reader.

The first chapter takes the reader through the purpose of assessment. The
reasons why assessment is so important in the education of students and
doctors are examined with parallels drawn with non-clinical examples. The
chapter goes on to describe the different aspects or dimensions of what we
are actually aiming to assess with the assessments we use. It ends with a
discussion around the meaning and implications of the terms 'competence',
'performance' and 'expert'.

The second chapter concentrates on the key principles of assessment and
covers terms that you are probably more familiar with such as validity and
reliability. Again, we offer some medical as well as non-medical examples
which we think will help with your understanding of these principles in
practice.

Chapter 3 considers the use of learning technologies which are moving at
a great pace in all fields of medical education, assessment is no different. New
forms of technology are not only helping with the administration of formative and summative assessments, but are also used in the construction of
specific individual tests tailored to students' needs and abilities.

Feedback is consistently mentioned by students and trainees as a problem.
Many learners do not recognise that feedback is given and often when feedback is provided, it is poorly structured with no relationship to the learning context. Feedback motivates improved performance, whether this is from
others or from yourself (through reflection). Opportunities to provide feedback are often wasted and many medical education assessors are particularly guilty of this. Chapter 4 explores the reasons behind these issues and
how teachers can develop ways of improving the giving and receiving of
feedback.

In Chapter 5, we look at portfolio assessments which are becoming
more commonplace within medical education. This is probably one area
of assessment that is viewed with the most cynicism by mature colleagues.
Like all forms of assessment it is only as good as its design and clarity of
purpose and structure. While little evidence exists around the impact on
learning of the tool, research has suggested that those trainees who are
unable or unwilling to complete portfolios have subsequent training issues
around professionalism.

Revalidation is a hot topic for all doctors. After passing our college exams doctors of a certain age certainly did not expect to be 'examined' again. We took part in our yearly appraisal, diligently presenting our gathered internal and external CPD points. Many doctors are worried about what revalidation is going to look like and the impact it will have on our practice. The final chapter sets out the GMC's current plans which to date do not look too much different from existing practices. However, for those of us in technical specialties, the spectre of simulation-based assessments is probably on the horizon.

Many different types of assessment are used in medical education in clinical and non-clinical settings and these are discussed in more detail in Chapters 7 and 8. In these chapters, the reader is guided through a discussion of each of these types, exploring how they are administered and their strengths and weaknesses. Chapter 9 discusses how these assessments are best combined into a coherent assessment programme.

For many educators, assessment brings one of the greatest challenges in teaching practice. It is when we are called to make judgements, not only on our learners but on the courses we teach and how we teach them. In writing this book, we are looking for ways this process can be made more enjoyable, effective, easier and more transparent.

We have purposefully not included a full bibliography with this text as there are many already in circulation and freely available to the reader, although we have provided some relevant references within each chapter. We believe that the glossary offered by the General Medical Council is a useful and thorough guide:

General Medical Council. *Glossary for the Regulation of Medical Education and Training*. Available from http://www.gmc-uk.org/GMC_glossary_for_medical_education_and_training.pdf_47998840.pdf (last accessed 3 October 2012)

Reference

1 Harden, R. Ten questions to ask when planning a course or curriculum. *Med Educ* 1986;**20**:356–65.

Chapter 1 **Purpose of assessment**

Learning outcomes

By the end of this chapter, you will be able to:
- Demonstrate an understanding of the purposes of assessment and why assessment is important
- Explain what we assess
- Demonstrate understanding of criterion and norm referencing
- Explain the terms competence, performance and expert

Assessment is often a source of considerable anxiety within the educational community as a whole, and the medical community is no exception. The aim of this chapter is to explore the rationale for and some of the key principles of assessment in the context of undergraduate, postgraduate and continuing medical education.

Assessment especially benefits from the coupling of theory with practice and the opportunity to develop 'an academic dialogue' [1]. However, it presents some challenges. As Cleland *et al.* [2] write:

> *[assessors need to] explore their (sometimes conflicting) roles as educators and assessors, and how they manage these roles, which are often conducted simultaneously in assessment situations.*

How to Assess Doctors and Health Professionals, First Edition. Mike Davis, Judy McKimm, and Kirsty Forrest.
© 2013 Blackwell Publishing Ltd. Published 2013 by Blackwell Publishing Ltd.

These tensions have increased with research and developments within educational assessment. Consequently, assessment has become more rigorous, systematic and objective. However, there is a potential gap between these developments and the role of clinicians, many of whom still think of their role in assessment as giving a subjective judgement of a one-to-one encounter.

Why do we assess?

The first question to ask is 'Why do we assess?' Before we go any further, consider the following scenarios:
- A cohort of first year undergraduates coming to the end of their first module in their degree programme.
- A cohort of final year undergraduates doing their finals (last exams).
- Students on a postgraduate distance learning programme who have completed all their taught modules and have to submit their dissertations before they graduate.
- Anaesthetic trainees attending a simulator centre who need to be signed off on their initial tests of competences prior to going on call.
- A group of doctors and nurses on a 3-day residential advance life support (ALS) resuscitation course.
- A group of physicians undertaking the membership examination.
- A surgeon submitting an MD thesis.

Why, in each of these scenarios, do you think there is need for assessment?

You might consider some or all of the following:
- Ensuring patient safety
- Predicting future behaviour
- Satisfying university requirements
- Judging level of learner achievement
- Monitoring learners' progress
- Motivating learners
- Measuring effectiveness of teaching
- Because they have pass to progress
- Professional/regulatory requirements
- Professional development
- Public expectations

There may be more than one reason for each scenario. On the other hand, not all reasons apply to all cases: for instance, the surgeon's MD would have little in common with an ALS course.

Activity 1.1

Please review and complete the following table, indicating (x) what you think are the reasons to assess in that situation:

	Undergraduate module exam in first year	Undergraduate finals examination	MSc dissertation	Simulation course	Resus course	Membership exam	MD thesis
Ensuring patient safety							
Predict future behaviour							
Judge level of learner achievement							
Monitor learner progress							
Motivate learners							
Measure effectiveness of teaching							
Public expectation							
Regulation (revalidation and/or recertification)							
Professional development							
Have to pass to progress							
University requirements							

Authors' completed version can be found on page 21.

Having completed the Activity 1.1, and reviewed the authors' completed version at the end of the Chapter, not all of these reasons are universally applicable. Let us look at some of these in more detail.

Ensuring patient safety

In certain contexts (e.g. work-based training and assessment) there is a close relationship between what a doctor does in managing a patient's case and the outcome for that patient. In other contexts, the relationship between trainees' actions and their impact on a potential patient is more tentative (e.g. the management of a case in a simulation suite cannot harm a real person but successful management in that setting might predict a competent performance on the ward). Assessment, therefore (i.e. passing or failing), is a potential proxy for good or bad outcomes in practice. A system that trains doctors and accredits them as being capable clinicians within an assessment regime is making an assumption that success in a simulated setting will transfer to clinical practice. We explore these issues later in the book.

Predicting future behaviour

The following extract illustrates the potential for uncertainty about the predictive nature of some assessments:

> The exam that really worked for me was the 11-plus. I was a very poor classroom performer and as a working-class student had no cultural springboard into education. It was a game-changer. That's the best thing I can say about the grammar school system – once I was at grammar school it was a different story. It was pure Darwinism – exams all the way. I was less keen on A-levels, as they coincided with the storms of adolescence and I did disastrously. I got two Cs and a D and had to go into the army. I eventually managed to get a place at Leicester University. Fortunately, it turned out to have a very good English Department. (John Sutherland, PhD, Emeritus Professor of English Literature [3])

For medicine, A-level grades are not a very good predictor of long-term student ability within medical school, especially in clinical settings. However, there is evidence that medical student grades in the first year of university are a very good predictor of future medical school grades.

Judging level of learner achievement

Both parties in the learning process are interested in the extent to which learners have achieved the outcomes set for them, whether for formative or summative purposes. The obvious example for medics is membership exams.

Monitoring learner progress

Informal, formative or ipsative (see Chapter 2 for more on these) assessment allows the outcomes from the assessment event to feed back into the learning process:

- Both parties need to know what is still to be done; where there are gaps in learner understanding or inaccurate perceptions
- To initiate remediation opportunities
- To determine ongoing programmes of study
- To feed into future sessional learning objectives and teaching plans
- To feed into curriculum review

This is often described as feedback and will be explored more thoroughly in Chapter 4. It can be in passing (informal), designed to improve performance (formative) and related to the learner's level (ipsative).

Motivating learners

The extent to which examinations motivate learners depends on the likely outcome. For some people, examinations can be highly demotivating – if they fail them. Take this quotation, for example:

> *I was never very good at exams, having a poor memory and finding the examination process rather artificial, and there never seemed to be enough time to follow up things that really interested me* [4]

Assessment can also be a driver for learning:

> *I am a big fan of exams. I think they're more meritocratic than coursework, especially at GCSE and A-level, when there's a lot of hot-housing by parents. I think stress can help bring out the best in you in an exam – there's something cleansing about it. I think we're far too averse to stress now. Exams are also good for teachers, as the last thing you want is continuing assessment. (Tristram Hunt, Lecturer in Modern British History* [3]*)*

Measuring effectiveness of teaching

Any course that has a significantly high failure rate has to look at a number of things, including the validity and reliability of its assessment regime, but also at the way in which it teaches the course or programme of study. A number of years ago, a Royal College took its membership examinations to the Indian sub-continent. The examination diet produced a 2% pass rate as candidates were almost completely out of their depth in the Objective Structured Clinical Examinations (OSCEs), never having experienced that teaching modality before. What the College had omitted to do was to prepare candidates to take the examination through a well-designed teaching programme.

Public expectation

While the public is less in awe of medical practitioners than once they were, they do have an expectation that doctors will know what to do and how to do it before they start to look after a group of patients. It is unlikely that they would be satisfied with the following notion:

> No physician is really good before he has killed one or two patients. (Hindu proverb [5])

Regulation (revalidation and/or recertification)

Issues related to revalidation are explored in Chapter 6.

Professional development

Continuing professional development can be seen as synonymous with learning and being fit to practice, and the assessment of its effectiveness is often the product of reflection and personal insight [6]. However, this is not considered by all to be adequate and revalidation is being introduced to address some of its limitations (see Chapter 6 for more on this).

Passing to progress/university requirements

Compare:

> The best joke question I ever saw was on the Basic Science final in Med School. One 4-hour exam on 2 years of material. It read: 'Given 1 liter of water, 10 moles of ATP and an Oreo cookie, create life. Show all formulas.' [7]

with:

> Back when I went to Oxford, the entrance exams for women were different. The one for Oxford I found most challenging was the general classics paper. It was a 3.5 hour paper – you had half an hour to think, then one hour for each question. I still remember one of the questions – 'compare the ideas of empire in Greece and Rome'. That was a real high jump intellectually. Exams are good things. They prepare you for later life with the stress and anticipation. (Susan Greenfield, Professor of Synaptic Pharmacology [3])

This sense of excitement and satisfaction is likely when candidates are successful, but what about this situation? On one occasion a student burst into his office. 'Professor Stigler, I don't believe I deserve this F you've given me.'

To which Stigler replied, '*I agree, but unfortunately it is the lowest grade the University will allow me to award.*'

While the experiences described above are different, motivation is a key component of what makes people succeed, sometimes despite the education system, not because of it. Motivation can be seen as extrinsic (stemming from outside the individual) or intrinsic (coming from within). Extrinsic motivators might include wanting to earn a better salary, achieve higher status or move to a higher level within the profession. Intrinsic motivators include achieving a feeling of personal satisfaction or wanting to learn more because something interests you rather than it being connected to career progression. While it is sometimes hard to separate the two, teachers need to work with learners to identify motivators, especially when students are struggling to pass assessments and are losing their sense of self-worth and achievement.

However, there is more to motivation and you have to consider the nature of examinees' responses to assessment events. Take, for example, the mathematics question shown in Figure 1.1.

3. Find x.

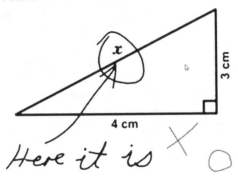

Figure 1.1 X marks the spot?

Clearly, the candidate is not motivated to 'find x' in the way in which the instruction expected.

> When revising for my primary membership exam (FRCA), I was learning about g-proteins and GABA receptors. These were new concepts to me but vitally important as this was how many of the anaesthetic drugs I gave worked within the human body. I pulled out my old pharmacology text book from medical school and turned to the relevant chapter. I found that I had previously underlined, at five separate times in five different colours while 'revising', these concepts. I

also found some old notes and saw that I was asked a written and viva question on this topic in the third MB pharmacology exam which I did quite well in. But I remembered absolutely nothing of it! (KF)

What are we assessing?

When assessing we need to link back to what we assume has been taught and learned, i.e. linking the assessment criteria to the learning objectives. The method of assessment must be appropriate to the relevant domain as well as to the context of learning in which the skill or behaviour has to be carried out.

You will have heard of the terms 'knowledge', 'skills' and 'attitudes'. These relate to the domains of learning first described by Bloom [8] in the 1950s to 1970s as the cognitive, psychomotor and affective domains, respectively. Effective clinical performance demands capability and performance in all three domains.

Traditionally, the elements required for a specific task have been taught in these separate domains. Using the task of a blood transfusion as an example: the knowledge basis of why a patient would need a transfusion is taught in lectures, e-learning or from books; the practical skills such as phlebotomy and cannulation are taught in skills laboratories or on the wards, the attitudinal or behavioural domains such as obtaining informed consent, explanation and counselling patients for transfusions are taught with simulated patients, role play, observation and in the workplace. The different ways of assessing these domains mirrors the way that we teach them.

Miller's pyramid (Figure 1.2) offers us another way to look at the progression of learning within a specific learning objective [9]. Miller's pyramid is often used for the assessment process to examine which level a learner has reached.

It may be helpful to think of this as a matrix:

Miller's pyramid stage	Teaching strategy	Assessment strategy	Example: blood transfusion
Does	Workplace	Performance/ competence	Performance (including affective domain)
Shows how	Simulation	OSCEs	Ditto above in training setting
Knows how	Skills lab	EMQs/vivas	Practical skills
Knows	Books, lectures	MCQs	How and when to transfuse

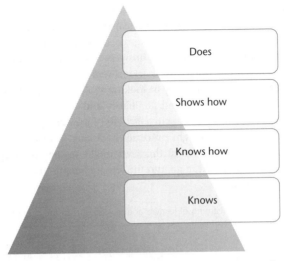

Figure 1.2 Miller's pyramid. Reproduced from [8] with permission from Wolters Kluwer Health.

What you will notice is that most assessment strategies do not tackle the tip of Miller's pyramid. We will explore more about this later.

The description of the division of learning into these three domains is over-simplistic and when looked at in more detail within each domain, a hierarchy of features becomes apparent; this is called a taxonomy. These levels are shown for each of the three learning domains in Table 1.1 [10].

Table 1.1 Taxonomies of learning

Cognitive, psychomotor and affective domains of learning from basic to advanced levels

Range of difficulty	Cognitive	Psychomotor	Affective
Basic	Knowledge	Perceiving	Receiving
	Comprehension	Patterning	Responding
	Application	Accommodation	Valuing
	Analysis	Refining	Organisation
	Synthesis	Improving	Characterisation
Advanced	Evaluation	Composing	

Data from Bloom [7] and Krathwohl *et al.* [10]).

The further up the hierarchy you go (see Table 1.2, Figure 1.3), the more complex the characteristics are of the feature, and therefore of the assessment; for example, knowledge, comprehension and application can be measured by MCQs or single word answers to questions. Application and analysis might lend themselves to short answers – two or three sentences. At the top of the hierarchy, you may be looking at a person's ability to respond to a prompt that would demand familiarity and comfort with knowledge from a number of fields of cognitive activity: for example, explorations of medico-legal work, or thought processes associated with complex clinical decision making. Assessment at this level might require an essay type of question so that learners can go into the required depth in order to explain their understanding.

Table 1.2 Definitions, learning objectives and assessments in the cognitive domain

The level of the hierarchy	Definition	Learning objective	Example: The assessment in relation to blood transfusion
Knowledge	Recall of information previously presented	Why do people bleed? What are the causes of anaemia?	MCQ, SAQ
Comprehension	Grasping the meaning but not extending it beyond the present situation	What levels of haemoglobin are acceptable	MCQ, SAQ
Application	Using the rules and principles	When would a patient require a transfusion	MCQ, SAQ, OSCE
Analysis	Breaking down components to clarify	Classify	OSCE
Synthesis	Arranging and assembling elements into a whole	How would you reduce the potential for future blood loss and requirements for transfusion?	OSCE, Viva, work-based place assessment (WBPA)
Evaluation	Ability to judge X for a purpose	When might a blood transfusion not be necessary	Viva, WBPA

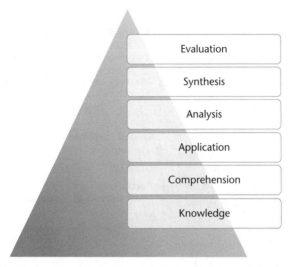

Figure 1.3 The cognitive domain. Reproduced from [9] with permission from Wolters Kluwer Health.

Questions can be helpful in assessing formatively (i.e. developmentally, not contributing to grades) where and how well the learner is operating in the cognitive domain.

An awareness of the cognitive levels can impact on the way in which questions are framed, Table 1.3.

Table 1.3 Levels of questioning within the cognitive domain

Level in domain	Focus	Example
Knowledge	Facts	What do A, B and C stand for in basic life support (BLS)?
Comprehension	What, why, when	Why does A come first?
Application	How?	When would you institute BLS on a street?
Analysis	Consequences?	What might the negative outcomes be?
Synthesis	Problem solving	How might you mitigate against the worst of these?
Evaluation	Planning for future design of intervention	What would impact on the design of a bystander BLS training programme?

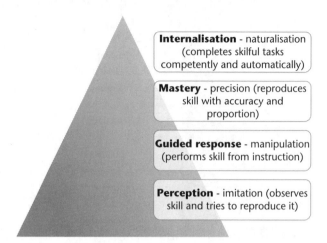

Internalisation - naturalisation (completes skilful tasks competently and automatically)

Mastery - precision (reproduces skill with accuracy and proportion)

Guided response - manipulation (performs skill from instruction)

Perception - imitation (observes skill and tries to reproduce it)

Figure 1.4 The psychomotor domain [11].

Teaching and learning methods for the psychomotor domain may well include some background knowledge (in this case some anatomy and physiology or running through the range of equipment needed), but for learners to perform this skill accurately, they need to practise. This may be on models or, with supervision and feedback, with patients. Assessment of competence would involve a number of observations, not simply asking the learner to describe what they would do.

In the simplified representation of the psychomotor domain shown in Figure 1.4, it will be evident that assessment opportunities are more appropriate at the higher levels: there would be little merit in formally assessing, for example, 'imitation' of a skill [11]. There could be value in making judgments about 'manipulation' as part of continuous assessment for the purposes of formative assessment but of greater value is summative assessment of complete skills at the level of 'precision'. This is the skill level where someone can demonstrate competence and the ability to function independently, but still has some way to go before having full autonomy with the related characteristics of expertise.

In our example of blood transfusion the skills necessary include phlebotomy, cannulation and prescribing. In the skills domain, the assessor's role is to observe (often with a structured checklist) and give feedback on performance. Ways of assessing can include: skills labs, OSCEs, or direct observation of procedures (DOPs).

In many respects, the affective domain presents the most difficulty in identifying clear assessment criteria as performance in this domain is so tied

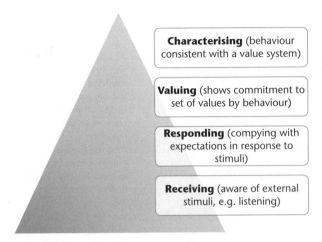

Figure 1.5 The affective domain.

up with subjective interpretations of behavioural data, only some of which is directly observable (Figure 1.5). For example, individuals manifest strong emotions in different ways and these are not always perceivable through what they say or do. So, for example, when an observer says 'You were angry in that consultation' that is describing a perceived emotion, but if the observer says 'You talked very quickly and loudly, glared at the patient and did not introduce yourself' these describe observable behaviours, not the underpinning emotional state.

In our blood transfusion example, the observable behaviours would include patient explanation and consent, acknowledging cultural or religious considerations in a non-judgemental way or counselling skills (listening, being empathic). Ways of assessing would include OSCEs, case-based discussion (CBD), mini clinical evaluation exercise (mini-CEX), objective structured long examination records (OSLERs), vivas or long cases.

As Epstein writes:

> *Dozens of scales that rate communication are used in medical education and research, yet there is little evidence that any one scale is better than another; furthermore, the experiences that patients report often differ considerably from ratings given by experts.* [12]

Despite this observation, efforts are made to assess for instructor candidacy based on affective characteristics such as these from the European Trauma Course (ETC), see Table 1.4 [13].

Table 1.4 Criteria for instructor candidates for European Trauma Course

Area	Basic criteria	Advanced criteria (with caveats)
Communication skills	Communicates effectively and appropriately; aware of audience	Active listener; recognises and uses subtleties in vocal factors in speech, such as tone of voice, tempo of speech; makes insightful comments; avoids redundancy and repetition
Commitment	Prepared for the course; full participation	Willingness to take on instructor responsibilities (may not be easy to show but may be demonstrated during informal discussion and mentoring sessions)
Credibility	Knowledgeable and able to communicate knowledge	Higher level perception, awareness and understanding in relation to ETC content and teaching method; able to contribute to ongoing developments; capacity for adding value to the course. May be demonstrated during informal discussions, feedback and mentoring sessions
Awareness of human factors	Recognises contribution of team members	Good interpersonal skills; able to get best from people as leader and member
Feedback	Insightful and accurate	Effective management and dialogue; willing to address complex issues

In the table above we show how the different elements of blood transfusion may be taught and assessed. However, this is an artificial representation of what actually happens in the workplace so there are drivers to change assessments to be more 'realistic' or authentic. This has led to the development of more 'integrated' assessments, where many elements of tasks are drawn together to test across a range of domains. These assessments would include OSLERs, longer OSCEs, long cases and vivas. For example, a learner might be asked to take a history from a patient who is tired all the time, provided with blood results showing anaemia, expected to counsel and obtain consent from the patient for a transfusion and prescribe the blood.

Becoming an expert

Looking back at Miller's pyramid, it implies through its hierarchy that a learner should have an appropriate knowledge base in order to be able to

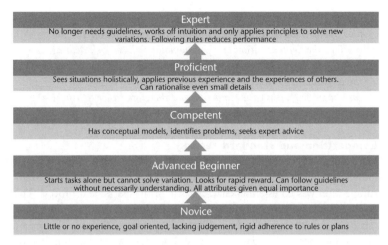

Figure 1.6 Novice to expert continuum.

perform a task competently. However, for some psychomotor skills, it is possible to 'do', without 'knowing' (certainly without knowing in depth); for example, the work of phlebotomists or bystanders using automatic defibrillators.

Miller's pyramid is often used to give a broad indication of the level a learner has reached, in order to identify appropriate learning strategies for the future. The model does not do justice to performance at higher levels (i.e. 'do') which might have varied levels of performance. This is examined through the final model to be explored in this chapter: the novice to expert continuum (Figure 1.6) developed by Dreyfus and Dreyfus [14].

Each of these levels has its own general criteria against which a person's performance can be judged. Clearly, a doctor or health professional could 'do' a procedure at a number of these levels, although competent is probably the level at which individuals might be thought capable of acceptable independent practice.

Traditionally, knowledge was the overriding domain that was taught and assessed in medical school and university. Practical skills were learned experientially (e.g. 'see one, do one, teach one') and new doctors and health professionals had to look to their seniors for examples or practice in the affective domain – often with unintended consequences, as this quote demonstrates:

> *Constructs such as professionalism have proven to be extraordinarily difficult to define, whereas constructs such as surgical procedures*

*appear much more amenable to definition. Generally, if a construct has
a component for which concrete quantitative measures are possible
(such as the demonstration of a psychomotor skill) or well-defined
indicator behaviours have been demonstrated as highly correlated to
the construct (such as selecting the correct diagnosis answer on a
case-based test), it is easier to define and therefore easier to assess
performance within the construct.* [15]

Competition and standard setting

Many doctors believe that their assessments were designed to compare one
individual with another. This, in the main, is now not the case. Historically,
competition was an essential characteristic of the assessment process. This
was a significant feature of public examinations (e.g. O and A-levels). Until
relatively recently public examinations were norm referenced. This meant
that the number of candidates who were allowed to pass an examination was
not dictated by the absolute standard that they achieved but by the number
of candidates who were allowed to pass. This was based on the application
of cut-off points on a normal distribution curve, depending on criteria that
may or may not relate to levels of achievement (Figure 1.7). The idea of
the competitive examination was introduced into British public life in
the middle of the nineteenth century to improve the quality of the British
civil service.

This simple yet powerful tool was used to manipulate the pass marks of
the results of examinations depending on issues of supply, for example, of

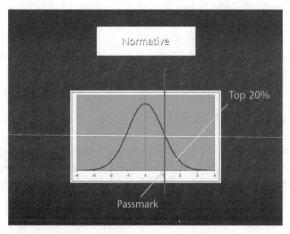

Figure 1.7 Normal distribution curve.

university places. This was a feature of UK higher education until 1963 when the post-Robbins reforms significantly expanded the number of university places available in the UK. Norm referencing was also used to manipulate the pass rate for entrance into medical Royal Colleges and has been introduced to allocate graduates to UK Foundation training posts.

Most educational institutions now use criterion referencing (see Activity 1.2). Criterion reference assessment can be likened to high jumping. The level of the bar is set and any learner who gets over the bar meets the criteria and passes. Assessment criteria are typically matched to the specified learning outcomes so that teaching, learning and assessment are all linked into one educational process.

Activity 1.2 Pros and cons of criterion and norm referencing

Think of both criterion and norm referencing – what advantages and disadvantages could be associated with these types of assessment process?

Criterion referenced: Pros	Cons

Norm referenced: Pros	Cons

Authors' completed version can be found on page 22.

Although there are advantages and disadvantages for each, the general behavioural differences produced are that norm referenced assessments produce a competitive atmosphere whereas criterion referenced assessment means that results of an assessment should be about the learner's achievement and not the assessment process itself.

Competence and performance

Aspiring to excellence

As with the completed Activity 1.2 at the end of the chapter, one of the disadvantages of criterion referencing is that learners might do just enough to pass. In 2007 an independent government inquiry was set up to look into the new postgraduate training scheme for medical doctors in the UK (Modernising Medical Careers). This was led by Sir John Tooke and its findings published in 2008 [16]. The report made a number of findings and recommendations. The first recommendation was as follows:

> *There must be clear shared principles for postgraduate medical training that emphasise flexibility and an aspiration to excellence.*

It had been recognised that much of medical education assessment was outcome or competency based, where the student who could achieve the competences was allowed to progress (both in undergraduate and postgraduate education). Criterion based methods of assessment may lend themselves to students learning to pass an examination rather than becoming a better healthcare professional. Using threshold competencies has led to a perception of a dumbing down of standards to the lowest common denominator. However, high achievers will always achieve. These forms of assessment do not always reward students for doing that little bit extra or 'aspiring to excellence' unless the assessments are carefully designed to enable and reward higher achievement and discriminate between candidates.

Competence is often described as only demonstrated in sterile environments (classrooms, skills labs, OSCEs), whereas performance is described as what someone would do in real life. However, competence can be seen as a point on the spectrum of performance (as in the Dreyfus model) which can be demonstrated in both the workplace and in simulated environments.

This concept is supported by the statement in Hager and Gonczi's [17] paper that all 'competency based assessments centre on performance'. There are some that even say performance is not 'real' either, because knowing that you are being observed changes your actions, known in social science as 'the Hawthorne effect'. The logical inference from this will be that the level of performance demonstrated in the simulated environments might not automatically translate into the same level of performance in the workplace.

You can see that the terms competence, competency and performance are often confused and clarification is needed when discussing the aims of an assessment.

Historically, we have tended to teach and assess in set patterns. Hodges [18] describes competence as being conceptualised in a variety of ways (or discourses), and if we emphasise one form of teaching and assessing over another we can actually create incompetence as a side-effect.

If we teach and assess in only one of these discourses, there is a danger of creating a one-dimensional doctor. Table 1.5 shows the four discourses and

Table 1.5 Discourses in competence

Discourse	Role of teacher	Role of student	Assessment measure	Hidden problems
Knowledge	Knowledge giver	Memorising and recall	MCQ and other short answer questions	Inability to recognise patterns; poor technical and interpersonal skills
Performance	Skills teacher	Practicing and demonstrating skills	Skills labs, simulations, OSCEs	Lack of integration of knowledge with performance; 'fake' performances
Reliable test score	Preparing students for standard assessments	Maximising scores on standardised measures	Standardised tests; OSCEs	Prolongation of novice behaviours; inability to deal with variation; lack of development of expert reasoning skills
Reflective practitioner	Guiding introspection; mentoring	Self-assessment and self-direction	Portfolio	Superficial self-assessment; development of reflective ability alone in the absence of knowledge and skills

the hidden problems that can arise if competence is emphasised in only one area. You may have noticed that these discourses follow an order of the chronological development of medical curricula and assessment methodologies. All the discourses have their pros and cons so contemporary assessment schemes combine all elements of these discourses.

Conclusions

What we have explored in this chapter is:
• An understanding of the purposes of assessment and why assessment is important
• What we assess
• An understanding of criterion and norm referencing
• Differences between competence and performance

There is some evidence to suggest that assessment drives learning, so if you want learners to know something, assess it. Think about your own experience. You have probably worked harder at learning something because it was going to be tested in some way. However, assessment has the capacity to encourage strategic learning (i.e. learning primarily to pass examinations) at the expense of deeper learning. This should not be seen in a negative light if there is a close relationship between the examination and levels of performance expected in clinical practice. Assessment design is therefore very important. Assessments must not only match the domain of learning (e.g. if you want to ensure competence in practice, a multiple choice examination about blood transfusions will not achieve that), but they must also work well in a practical sense and encourage learners to apply their knowledge to increasingly complex situations. In this way, assessments help learners to move along the 'novice to expert' continuum as they start to integrate knowledge, skills and attitudes/behaviours within their clinical practice.

For the clinical teacher, working with students or trainees in everyday clinical situations, it is sometimes hard to see the way in which the assessments you are involved relate to the wider university or training context and assessment theory. However, the principles underpinning effective assessment apply in a wide range of contexts and it is to these that we turn next.

Activity 1.1 Authors' version of the reasons for assessment by scenario table seen earlier in this chapter

	Undergraduate module exam in first year	Undergraduate finals examination	MSc dissertation	Simulation course	Resus course	Membership exam	MD thesis
Ensuring Patient safety		X		X?	X		
Predict future behaviour	X	X	X	X	X		X
Judge level of learner achievement	X	X	X		X	X	
Monitor learner progress	X		X	X	X		
Motivate learners	X	X	X	X	X		X
Measure effectiveness of teaching	X	X	X	X	X		X
Public expectation		X				X	
Regulation (revalidation and/or recertification)				X	X	X	
Professional development			X	X		X	X
Have to pass to progress	X	X				X	
University requirements	X	X	X				X

Activity 1.2 Authors' version of the pros and cons of criterion and norm referencing

Criterion referenced: Pros	Cons
Criteria are known by students, therefore they know what they have to revise and learn to pass	Students might learn only the bare minimum and not engage with wider aspects of the programme
Sets minimum performance expectations	Hard to set the standard, could be too low or too high, adjusted for local demand
Demonstrates what students can and cannot do in relation to the standards – competency based	If the standard is sufficiently well known within a target community, there may be a temptation to aspire only to pass rather than to surpass that standard, thereby encouraging a culture of mediocrity

Norm referenced: Pros	Cons
Ensures a spread across the group	Top and bottom performances can be very close in groups of similar ability
Shows student performance across the group	Dispenses with absolute criteria for performance. Being above average does not necessarily imply a great performance
Useful to identify specific numbers of passes for limited places	Variation year on year or between exams can lead to challenges of inequity and unfairness

References

1 Ringsted C, Henriksen A, Skaarup M and van der Vleuten, C. Educational impact of in-training assessment (ITA) in postgraduate medical education: a qualitative study of an ITA programme in actual practice. *Med Educ* 2004;**38**:767–77.
2 Cleland J, Knight L, Rees C, Tracey S and Bond C. Is it me or is it them? Factors that influence the passing of underperforming students. *Med Educ* 2008;**42**, 800–9.
3 Batty D. My exam nightmare: views from academia. *The Guardian*, **13** July 2009.
4 Paul Nurse. BrainyQuote.com, Xplore Inc, 2011. Available at: http://www.brainyquote.com/quotes/quotes/p/paulnurse292730.html (accessed 3 October 2012).
5 Hindu proverb. Available at: http://www.quotegarden.com/experience.html (accessed 3 October 2012).

6 Schostak J, Davis M, Hanson J, Schostak J, Brown T, Driscoll P, *et al.* 'Effectiveness of Continuing Professional Development' Project: a summary of findings. *Med Teach* 2010;**32**:586–92.

7 http://www.freerepublic.com/focus/f-chat/2291437/posts (accessed 3 October 2012).

8 Bloom B. *Taxonomy of Educational Objectives. Handbook I: The cognitive domain.* New York: David McKay Co Inc, 1956.

9 Miller G. The assessment of clinical skills, competence, performance. *Acad Med* 1990;**65**:S63–7.

10 Krathwohl D, Bloom B and Masia B. *Taxonomy of Educational Objectives, the classification of educational goals. Handbook II: The affective domain.* New York: David McKay Co Inc, 1973.

11 Simpson E. *The Classification of Objectives in the Psychomotor Domain.* Washington DC: Gryphon House, 1972.

12 Epstein R. Assessment in medical education. *N Engl J Med* 2007;**356**:387–96.

13 European Trauma Course (ETC). *Instructor potential assessment.* Internal ETC document, 2009.

14 Dreyfus H and Dreyfus S. *Mind over Machine: the power of human intuition and expertise in the era of the computer.* Oxford: Basil Blackwell, 1986.

15 Andreatta P and Gruppen L. Conceptualising and classifying validity evidence for simulation. *Med Educ* 2009;**43**,1028–35.

16 Tooke J. Aspiring to excellence. Available at: http://www.mmcinquiry.org.uk/Final_8_Jan_08_MMC_all.pdf (accessed 7 October 2012).

17 Hager P and Gonczi A. What is competence? *Med Teach* 1996;**18**:15–8.

18 Hodges B. Medical education and the maintenance of incompetence. *Med Teach* 2006;**28**:690–6.

Chapter 2 **Principles of assessment**

Learning outcomes

By the end of this chapter, you will be able to:
- Demonstrate an understanding of some of the principles of assessment including validity, reliability, specificity, feasibility and fidelity
- Demonstrate an understanding of the difference between formal and informal assessment
- Demonstrate an understanding of the difference between formative and summative assessment and the impact of high, medium and low stakes assessment
- Identify opportunities for the longitudinal assessment of performance

When designing and conducting assessments, a number of key principles need to be considered. Each of these principles has an impact on the trustworthiness of an assessment.

Validity

In general terms, validity is the measure of the truthfulness of the assessment. In other words, does the assessment have a close relationship to the 'real world' phenomena that it is seeking to replicate? From this perspective, the most valid assessment would be one conducted entirely within the context of a real event or series of events. For example, a driving test would be a real

How to Assess Doctors and Health Professionals, First Edition. Mike Davis, Judy McKimm, and Kirsty Forrest.
© 2013 Blackwell Publishing Ltd. Published 2013 by Blackwell Publishing Ltd.

journey between two locations that would involve the full spectrum of driving conditions that a learner might expect to meet:

- Town centre
- Motorway
- Driving faster than 30 mph
- Adverse weather conditions
- Other drivers

Similarly, the ability to manage a patient with chest pain would be assessed during the management of a real patient in the actual place that this would occur, the acute medical admission unit, with the team of people and equipment that would be there. If you add in all conditions that a learner might expect to meet these could include the following:

- Non-English speaking patient
- Chest pain worsening
- Oxygen cylinder emptying

Obviously, you can see how this cannot be done routinely and, while not impossible, would make enormous demands on resources to be effective. Work-based assessment is one way that we can get close to this and this will be covered in later chapters.

Classic views of validity explain this in terms of the content of an assessment, the criteria used and the constructs the assessment is trying to measure. Reliability (reproducibility) of an assessment is seen as a separate test trait and measured separately. More contemporary views suggest that all validity is construct validity, that scientific measurements need to be applied to tests (to provide evidence) and that reliability is part of validity [1–3]. Below we explain the classic views of assessment as these are still in common usage, and include some of the more recent perspectives where relevant.

To ensure validity we need to provide evidence on the purpose, intended interpretation and meaning of the assessment and to seek multiple sources of scientific evidence. The higher the stakes of the assessment, the more evidence is required. So, in the classic view, for an assessment to be valid it has to meet a number of conditions.

Content validity

If an assessment has content validity, it is testing those phenomena that accurately reflect the real world. Look, for example, at these three questions from an imaginary philosophy examination:

1. What were the circumstances of Socrates' death?
2. What is the meaning of 'Cogito, ergo sum?'
3. Why?

What were the circumstances of Socrates' death?

Socrates was executed in Athens in 399 BCE after being found guilty of corrupting minors. He could have avoided death but he refused to accept banishment as an alternative punishment.

What needs to be considered here is the knowledge domain that is being tested and how that relates to that body of knowledge that is artificially conceived of as 'philosophy'. The important thing here is that a student does not need to have any understanding of Socrates' contribution to knowledge to answer this question successfully. As knowledge, this question might fit more accurately into a history examination or as an item of trivia in a pub quiz.

Accordingly, this would not meet the criteria for content validity for the philosophy examination.

What is the meaning of 'Cogito, ergo sum?'

This question looks more promising. It contains the famous Cartesian maxim, and it appears to be intent on exploring meaning, which in itself is a concern of philosophy. However, there is an answer that demands no understanding of philosophy:

A: 'I think, therefore I am.'

While this is correct – i.e. an accurate translation of the phrase – the answer does nothing to uncover the intention behind Descartes' maxim, which was to explore the ontological proof of the existence of God. At its most simplistic, the question, as it stands, is an invitation to translate something from Latin and a candidate could be 'correct' without showing any evidence of understanding Descartes' philosophy.

Why?

This question apocryphally appeared in a Cambridge philosophy examination and the answer that supposedly obtained a starred first was 'Why not?'
Explanations for this vary:
- An intelligent answer to a stupid question
- A stupid answer to an intelligent question
- A stupid answer to a stupid question
- An intelligent answer to an intelligent question

Or, more mundanely, a wry commentary on the sciolism (superficial knowledge) of academia (courtesy of [4]).

In each of these three cases, the content of the assessment might appear to be one thing, but it is, in fact, another. Question 3, 'Why?', might be an exception to this, but it is unlikely.

You might be able to think of examples of this type of mismatch from your own experiences of being examined.

Face validity
All the questions above might, however, seem to be appropriate. What they have is face validity. In other words, they look as if they might be testing what they set out to test. They occupy the relevant knowledge domain, use appropriate language, are framed in a subject relevant way and, at first glance, might seem to be appropriate. In this sense, face validity is the easiest criterion for an assessment item to meet.

Examples of this might be MCQ (true/false) questions such as these, from the Advanced Paediatric Life Support Course VLE [5]:
1. A child in ventricular asystole is rarely acidotic
   a. True
   b. False
2. A child in ventricular asystole should be given 10 μg/kg adrenaline (epinephrine) as the first drug
   a. True
   b. False

Predictive validity
This measure of an assessment item has, in some respects, the most serious implications within the context of medical education. It poses the question: 'Would success in this activity imply similar success if these conditions were met in, for example, a resuscitation room.' Objective structured clinical examinations (OSCEs) and other simulated scenario based assessments are good examples of activities that, it would be hoped, accurately reflect the real world. The assumption underlying this criterion is that if a candidate can demonstrate appropriate knowledge, skills and attitudes in the examination context, then the same level of performance could be expected in real clinical practice. However, compare the following:

> Correlating assessment with future performance is difficult not only because of inadequacies in the assessment process itself but also because relevant, robust measures of outcome that can be directly attributed to the effects of training have not been defined [6]

with:

> The OSCE examination tests a wide range of skills thus greatly reducing the sampling error. This very significantly improves the reliability of the examination. [7]

Reliability

Reliability explores the extent to which the results of an assessment are an accurate and consistent measurement of a candidate's demonstration of abilities as specified in assessment criteria. These criteria can be general (i.e. they could apply to any set of circumstances) or specific (i.e. they relate to a particular set of conditions). There are three key words in this definition:

1. criteria
2. accurate
3. consistent

Assessment criteria (as they relate to cognitive and affective domains and, to a lesser extent, the psychomotor domain) can be very straightforward or very complex and, by definition, any point in between, depending on the level of knowledge being assessed. You may need to remind yourself of the hierarchies introduced briefly in Chapter 1.

To explore this complexity, consider the answer schemes to the following questions.

Question	Answer/assessment criteria
Q1. What year was the Battle of Hastings?	1066
Q2. Consider your experiences of online communities. To what extent do they replicate experiences face to face? Do you consider that online communities can be characterised as being 'fragmented by technologies'? [8]	*Upper second (60–69)*: An essay meriting an upper second mark displays an ability to handle the relevant literature and research in a critical and analytical matter. It is more than a good description of the various theories, studies and perspectives relevant to the question. It does not necessarily have a watertight argument, but it is clearly structured and its conclusion does not take the reader by surprise. An upper-second essay develops a well-expressed theme or argument from a critical and appropriately referenced consideration of relevant literature. Competing claims, and the evidence advanced in defence of them, are examined and evaluated. An upper-second essay avoids unsubstantiated assertions.

There are a number of differences that are immediately recognisable. There is a single 'right' answer to Q1. While mathematicians, accountants and statisticians might quibble about the meaning of 1066 as a number, there is a shared interpretation of it ('ten sixty-six') as a calendar year, even without the AD or CE suffix.

Q2 on the other hand, poses some problems. In choosing either general or specific criteria as assessment tools, the examiner is determining whether there is an intention to have a particular answer in mind, or one that allows the candidate a degree of flexibility and choice in how to answer the question. General criteria are often employed where a question is sufficiently open to interpretation. More specific criteria are employed when examiners want candidates to demonstrate an understanding of specific issues. Consider the following as an example of specific criteria for an examiner:

> *The candidate provides an accurate and reasonably detailed description of a difference between Short Term Memory (STM) and Long Term Memory (LTM) that demonstrates relevant knowledge and understanding. For example, the candidate has clearly described a difference such as different durations and has described the durations of STM as being up to 30 seconds in duration and LTM as being potentially life long in reasonable detail. The difference does not have to be separately/explicitly identified to attract the full 3 marks as long as the description makes the difference clear* [9].

An example for a short answer question from the fellowship of the Royal College of Anaesthetists' exam goes some way to explaining how the question will be marked:

> *What are the important organisational (40%) and clinical (50%) considerations that govern the anaesthetic management of patients with morbid obesity? 10% of the marks for each question will be awarded for clarity, judgment and the ability to prioritise; marks will be deducted for serious errors.*

Both accuracy and consistency are essential characteristics of an assessment if that assessment is to have any currency beyond the event itself. Failure of an assessment to meet this essential condition leads an examination system to be thought of as unfair.

If appropriate criteria have been met in the design of an examination scheme, reliability can fail as a consequence of inadequate training, preparation and support of examiners. Assessment systems have an obligation to guarantee this. Accordingly, most programmes of assessment have rigorous preparation sessions for both experienced and new examiners. As well as spelling out general obligations (e.g. not favouring certain candidates), this training is important in helping to ensure that all examiners would reach the same decision given the same response. In some cases, this is quite straightforward. Consider:

Q. What year was the Battle of Hastings? Circle a, b or c.
   a. 1066
   b. 1215
   c. 1914–1918

The answer is, as we all know, a. This approach to testing 'knowledge' (see Chapter 1 for its place in the cognitive hierarchy) is easy and can by managed by machine – either computers or optical readers can be used to mark even complex multiple choice examinations.

However, even something a little more complex adds more difficulty. Consider:

Q. What year was the Battle of Hastings? Write in your answer in the blank space below.
   A.

In this case, the respondent's open answer has to be read and interpreted by a human agency or by a much more sophisticated computer programme than that used to mark multiple choice answers.

However, if the question wanted to ask a much more complex question (i.e. further up the cognitive hierarchy), the responses would have to be judged by people with subject expertise and appropriate training.

The examiners for these assessments would need to be subject experts and they would need to agree on the result of an assessment, given the same evidence from the same assessment event. This is very easy in the case of the year of the Battle of Hastings. At worst, the judgement might be that:

1066 CE

is the same as

Ten sixty-six

or another representation of the same date.

NB. If the assessment criteria for the above question were refined, however, to include the words 'using conventional criteria for depicting dates' then only the first answer would be acceptable.

While this is more complicated the more difficult the question is, at least in a written answer, there is the opportunity to check the application of the assessment criteria and subject a decision to critical analysis, or, at its simplest, agreement trials or some other kind of multiple marking. This is much more difficult if the assessment event is some kind of 'live' event: an OSCE, a simulation or a work-based learning activity. In this case (unless the event is being video recorded) the examiner has to rely on complex variables:

- Perception of events in order
- The accuracy of perception

For this reason, it is not unusual in formal events (like OSCEs in membership or fellowship examinations) for there to be two examiners.

The presence of two examiners raises one of two related issues: inter-rater and intra-rater reliability. Inter-rater reliability describes the condition that exists when two examiners, seeing an identical performance, would come to the same opinion as to a mark or a pass/fail assessment. The challenge, in this case, is in the perception of events as they unfold in real time. Consider the following simulation scenario assessment conducted during an ALS course (or similar):

A 22-year-old man is brought into emergency department. It is obvious that he has been in a fight and he is slightly drunk. During the management of airway and breathing it is noticed that blood is pooling on the trolley. A log roll reveals a deep knife wound in the lower back.

There are at least three views of what the assessed person was doing during this simulation:

1. What actually happened
2. What examiner 1 saw
3. What examiner 2 saw

There is a considerable body of literature on 'eye-witness testimony', particularly in the context of reconstructive memory, as in this account of the work of Bartlett:

Bartlett's theory of reconstructive memory is crucial to an understanding of the reliability of eyewitness testimony as he suggested that recall is subject to personal interpretation dependent on our learnt or cultural norms and values – the way we make sense of our world.

Many people believe that memory works something like a videotape. Storing information is like recording and remembering is like playing back what was recorded, with information being retrieved in much the same form as it was encoded. However, memory does not work in this way. It is a feature of human memory that we do not store information exactly as it is presented to us. Rather, people extract from information the gist, or underlying meaning [10].

In other words, people store information in the way that makes the most sense to them. This can be likened to a computer where there is information input, storage and retrieval. From this perspective, depending on how information is presented and understood by learners (who might all store this in different 'directories' with different labels) their ability to retrieve meaningful information varies. This is why we categorise information under various labels such as 'physiology', heart failure' or the 'renal system'. Another view suggests that we make sense of information by trying to fit it into schemas, which are a way of organising information. Schemas are mental 'units' of knowledge that correspond to frequently encountered people, objects or situations. They allow us to make sense of what we encounter in order that we can predict what is going to happen and what we should do in any given situation. This is very relevant to clinical learning. These schemas may, in part, be determined by social values and therefore can be prejudiced.

Schemas are therefore capable of distorting unfamiliar or unconsciously 'unacceptable' information in order to 'fit in' with our existing knowledge or schemas. This can, therefore, result in unreliable eyewitness testimony. [10]

This is supplemented by any other observers (nurses, assisting doctors) and by the actor playing the patient. Contemporary theories consider that multiple sources of evidence are needed to make reliable judgements. This might be over time (so that students are assessed on the same construct on multiple occasions and contexts) or by multiple raters, such as in multi-source feedback (explored further in Chapter 5). The higher the stakes, the more evidence from multiple sources is required.

The focus thus far has been on inter-rater reliability and we need also to consider intra-rater reliability (i.e. the capacity for an individual to make consistent judgements over time). This can be affected by a number of factors, including the following:

- Tiredness (e.g. after a long day of OSCE assessments in a fellowship examination)
- A possible existing relationship between examiner and examinee
- Lack of clarity or precision in the marking scheme or assessment schedule

Let us consider these in turn.

Tiredness

Many examination regimes make great demands on examiners and their capacity to maintain concentration over long periods of time and the impact on this might include the following:

- Inattention
- Boredom
- Irritation

all leading to inconsistent application of criteria.

Inappropriate relationships

Any relationship between examiners and examinees can distort the process and efforts have been made to discourage inappropriate relationships particularly. What follows is not untypical guidance from an American university:

> *Faculty members exercise power over students, whether in giving them praise or criticism, evaluating them, making recommendations for their further studies or their future employment, or conferring any other benefits on them. All amorous or sexual relationships between faculty members and students are unacceptable when the faculty member has any professional responsibility for the student. Such situations greatly increase the chances that the faculty member will abuse his or her power and sexually exploit the student. Voluntary consent by the student in such a relationship is suspect, given the fundamental asymmetric nature of the relationship. Moreover, other students and faculty may be affected by such unprofessional behaviour because it places the faculty member in a position to favour or advance one student's interest at the expense of others and implicitly makes obtaining benefits contingent on amorous or sexual favours. [11]*

The implication here is that an examinee who has a relationship with an examiner will somehow benefit from that relationship (the halo effect) but there is a great deal of informal evidence to suggest that this is not the case: that students, for example, in higher education who have relationships with their tutors, get lower grades in assessments and examinations. Either way, it is clear that this can distort the assessment process and should be avoided where possible. Where it is not possible – work-based assessment can be an example of this – the implications need to be made as open as possible. We can help to increase intra-rater and inter-rater reliability by training, feedback, using multiple assessors, clear marking schemes and robust moderation methods.

Lack of clarity in marking scheme

Many marking schemes are the product of considerable discussion and debate and it is right that they should be. However, this can lead to a lack of clarity and the potential for a variety of interpretations to be put on them. This is particularly true the further up any of the domain hierarchies the assessment event is addressing – hence some of the challenges associated with revalidation, to be explored in Chapter 6.

Most marking schemes are the product of an iterative process designed to test their robustness. This includes conducting assessment trials and making close examination of results to see if the assessment scheme throws up any statistical anomalies. By the time a scheme is being applied in a real examination setting, it should be robust and any variation in application could be the product of intra-rater reliability (i.e. the product of inconsistent marking by an individual examiner). The presence of second examiners in many face to face contexts, and second markers in written examinations can mitigate against the worst effect of this.

Specificity

There are many cases, particularly in the context of something as complex as the practice of medicine, in which it is important to assess the ability to meet certain practical criteria within their normal context. The challenge for the assessment designer is to ensure that the knowledge, skill or attitude being assessed is not buried in a mountain of other, non-assessed components.

One particular issue that is specific to medicine is the concept of 'case specificity'. A candidate may perform well in a single encounter with a patient; however, this does not mean that they would perform equally well with another patient with the same complaint or a completely different condition. This has been the driving force that has moved away from long case examinations and towards the OSCE examination where candidates must perform well in a large number of patient presentations. The same is true of written cases and, similarly, this has driven medical assessment away from essays towards shorter question formats which allow the testing of multiple domains of knowledge and much wider sampling of the learning outcomes that need to be tested. Here, blueprinting the assessments against all the learning outcomes in a programme helps to ensure that sufficient test items are included to sample widely across all domains of knowledge, skills and behaviours.

In terms of practical skills, inserting a cannula as part of the management of circulation in a resuscitation algorithm of airway, breathing and circulation can be demonstrated within the context of a case (i.e. in a scenario or simulation). It also can be demonstrated as a discrete skill within a clinical skills laboratory. If the target skill is only cannula insertion, it would be inappropriate to begin an examination scenario at the initial assessment and end it with arrangements for transfer to the ICU. It would be sufficient to contextualise the skill briefly within a short clinical case.

Many 'new' designers of simulation cases have a tendency to write the scenarios with non-specific criteria in mind. This is usually crystallised and reviewed when they pilot their cases.

Specifically, specificity means that you test what you mean to test.

Feasibility

Feasibility changes over time and is very much dependent on time, culture, innovation and finance. Teaching and assessing breast examinations on consenting patients was considered the norm in the 1980s. It was affordable, possible and appropriate. With changing social values and patient expectations and the development of realistic clinical skills manikins the use of these has become routine and suggestions of using patients for initial teaching is met with looks of disbelief.

OSCEs were originally thought to be unfeasible because of the logistics and cost of running them and now they are present in most undergraduate and postgraduate assessments.

What this means for assessments within medical contexts is that they have to be possible given the resource limitations and their implications. As we will be exploring when we look at fidelity later, while it would be extremely valid to assess, for example, extraction at a major road traffic collision on the M6 outside Stoke, it would not be feasible to do so for so many reasons. For practical, ethical and organisational reasons it would not be possible to rely on the occurrence of real events for the purposes of assessment.

Feasibility, therefore, is a challenge to fidelity.

Fidelity

What this has led to over a number of years is the use of simulations of varying design and complexity. Regardless of any constraints, the designs have always striven to be faithful reproductions of real events. This has been achieved, to a large extent, to be the product of one of two stage illusions:

1. 'Sleight of hand', where the magician leads the audience to see what he wants them to see.

2. 'The willing suspension of disbelief', where the audience buys into the notion that what they see on the stage or the screen is really happening in front of their eyes.

Among the consequences of this is that participants in simulated events, whether teaching or assessment, can buy into the reality of a case even though they are aware that it is a simulation. Issenberg *et al.* [12] concluded that fidelity was one of the predictors for high quality simulation that is educationally effective.

Formal and informal assessment: assessment of learning as opposed to assessment for learning

Thinking about whether an assessment is of learning or for learning is an important consideration when considering the nature and intentions behind formal and informal assessment. As van der Vleuten and Schuwirth write:

> *The weights attached to the criteria in a very high stakes assessment, for instance a certifying examination, will be very different from the distribution of weights among the criteria when the primary purpose of the assessment is to provide feedback to students in an in-training context. [13]*

A useful way of thinking about the difference between a formal and an informal assessment is to compare a driving test with a driving lesson. In the former, the candidate is put in a number of typical situations and is expected to perform to a standard that is safe and, to a degree, confident. Usually, at this stage, the candidate has achieved the level of 'mastery' in the psycho-motor domain. In effect, the learner driver is being exposed to a simulated version of normal urban driving, and the performance is being judged against a set of criteria. While these are not made explicit to the candidate during the test, they should be well known, largely as a product of a systematic training programme and the candidate's perceptions of what it means to be a driver.

At the end of the test, the examiner makes a decision on the basis of these criteria and candidates are either told that they have passed the test or that they have failed to meet some specific criteria and they have to be tested again.

During a lesson, on the other hand, the instructor is still making judgements about the candidate's ability to meet criteria but these do not trigger the final pass/fail assessment. This does not mean, however, that those assessments do not have any benefit to either the candidate or the instructor. They are informal but they have a considerable value in making judgements about students' progress and to a certain extent predicting future performance, while at the same time, identifying opportunities for development.

Formal assessment, then, is often an event while informal assessment is a process and this lends itself, therefore, to being a mechanism for assessing affect and other human factors related behaviours.

Formative and summative assessment

This same analogy can be used to pursue the difference between formative and summative assessment. This dimension is different in character to the informal–formal one described earlier. The informal nature of assessment of performance in the driving lesson is to provide information for the purposes of review and (it is to be hoped) subsequent improved performance. As such, it has a formative process in that it is going to lay the basis for feedback about performance; this is assessment for learning. These types of assessment are low and medium stakes. High stakes assessments are summative and focused on assessment of learning. Typically, many finals or licencing examinations do not provide detailed feedback to learners, just a grade or pass mark.

The two dimensions of formal and informal and formative and summative can be brought together in this matrix in the context of learning to drive:

	Informal	Formal
Formative	General impressions of psychomotor and skills performance	Awareness of highway code (e.g. mini-quiz; computer based test)
Summative	Final driving lesson before test	Driving test

and more generally;

	Informal	Formal
Formative	Observation	Practice assessment
Summative	Continuous or outcome based assessment	Final examination at university

---

Activity 2.1 Your experiences

Think about some contexts closer to medical education. How might you complete this matrix? See the end of the chapter for some possible responses.

	Informal	Formal
Formative		
Summative		

Authors' completed version can be found on page 39.

Ipsative assessment

Ipsative assessment can be formal or informal, and formative but not summative, and it is located in recognition of change in a person's performance over time. In other words, ipsative assessment identifies the extent to which an assessee has improved between assessment episodes. In this case, there is no reference to external characteristics (i.e. neither norms nor criteria – see Chapter 1). An example of this might be the way in which an athlete's performance improves over time. In the clinical setting, ipsative assessment is more likely to be a feature of work-based assessment where a trainee may be given increasingly difficult skills to practise and manage, as confidence, knowledge and dexterity grow.

Continuous assessment

Continuous assessment is used to describe the longitudinal assessment of performance of an individual. It is a process rather than an event and is designed to take some of the pressure out of consideration of a person's competence. Surprisingly, despite the widespread recognition that it allows candidates to perform to a higher standard, it is often thought of as an easier option and one that does not test candidates' capacity in the same way as formal summative assessments. The debate about coursework versus final examinations at both school and university is illustrative of this and at the time of writing we are seeing the pendulum swing back to assessing A-levels by final examination rather than using course work.

While this debate continues, continuous assessment has another widespread manifestation: the use of portfolios, which are examples of continuous self-assessment, where trainees record their own achievements over time.

Conclusions

These principles of assessment can be in competition with one another. Consider this:

You are in charge of assessing a whole year of fourth year medical students in their ability to pass a urinary catheter. The gold standard way this could be done would be by observing a student performing the procedure on a patient. This would be definitely valid, have specificity and fidelity, might be reliable, if we believe that what we see that day would be repeated another day, but not very feasible for many different reasons.

This challenge is often called the utility equation.

The utility of an assessment was defined as a product of its reliability, validity, cost-effectiveness, acceptability and educational impact [14]:

$$\text{The usefulness of an assessment} = \text{educational impact} \times \text{reliability} \times \text{validity} \times \text{cost effectiveness} \times \text{acceptability}$$

While the equation does not include all aspects of assessments, it serves as a reminder of the different aspects involved with planning assessment strategies for a single assessment or a whole curriculum. Each of these principles of assessment make competing claims on the design of the event and concessions have to be made, usually in descending order of presentation here. In other words, for practical reasons, it is more likely that fidelity will be sacrificed to reliability.

Activity 2.1 Your experiences – possible responses

	Informal	Formal
Formative	Observation (e.g. of skills or affect) on placement	Practice OSCE
Summative	Recommendation for instructor status; observation of work-based practice (DOPS)	Fellowship examination

References

1 Cronbach LJ. Five perspectives on validity argument. In Wainer H and Braun H (Eds). *Test Validity*. Hillsdale, NJ: Lawrence Erlbaum, 1988, pp. 3–17).

2　Messick S. Validity. In Linn RL (Ed.) *Educational Measurement*, 3rd edn. Washington, DC: The American Council on Education and the National Council on Measurement in Education, 1989, pp. 13–103.

3　Kane MT. Validation. In Brennan RL (Ed.) *Educational Measurement*, 4th edn.) Washington, DC: The National Council on Measurement in Education and the American Council on Education, 2006, pp. 17–64.

4　Why ask why? Available at: http://www.snopes.com/college/exam/oneword.asp (accessed 7 October 2012).

5　ALSG. APLS Pre-course VLE, 2011. Available at: http://www.alsg.org/vle/mod/quiz/attempt.php?id=48708 (accessed 4 October 2012).

6　Epstein MD. Assessment in Medical Education. In Ronald M and Epstein MD. *N Engl J Med* 2007;**356**:387–96.

7　Harden RM. What is an OSCE? *Med Teach* 1988;**10**:19.

8　Lancaster University Department of Educational Research Psychology in Education 301. *Assessment criteria.* Internal document, 2009.

9　AQA. GCE Mark Scheme, 2006 January series. *Psychology A.*

10　McLeod S. Eyewitness testimony, 2009. Available at: http://www.simplypsychology.org/eyewitness-testimony.html (accessed 4 October 2012).

11　Indiana University Academic Handbook (1997. Available at: http://enrollmentbulletin.indiana.edu/pages/consent.php?Term=2 (accessed 4 October 2012).

12　Issenberg SB, McGaghie WC, Petrusa ER, Lee Gordon D and Scalese, R. Features and uses of high-fidelity medical simulations that lead to effective learning: a BEME systematic review. *Med Teach* 2005;**27**:10–28.

13　van der Vleuten CPM and Schuwirth LWT. Assessing professional competence: from methods to programmes. *Med Educ* 2005;**39**:309–17.

14　van der Vleuten CPM. The assessment of professional competence: developments, research and practical implications. *Adv Health Sci Educ* 1996;**1**:41–67.

Chapter 3 E-assessment – the use of computer-based technologies in assessment

> **Learning outcomes**
>
> By the end of this chapter you will be able to:
> - Recognise the scope and impact of technology in the development of assessment and feedback
> - Describe the use of computer-based technology in the delivery of assessments
> - Identify the possibilities that computer technology offer for assessments in your area
> - Recognise the advantages and disadvantages of using computers for different assessment modalities

Many changes have been made over recent years in using computer-based technologies for assessments, evaluation and feedback. For many of us, assessments in our medical training involved little or no computer-based technology. The idea of a fairer, more objective way of being examined is very attractive compared to the perceived hawkish viva or long case examiner. However, we must be wary that just because the technology is available, does not mean we have to use it. Often it is easy to forget that the technology used in assessments should support learners' needs.

Technology can be very useful when used in assessment, evaluation and feedback, especially when learners are dispersed, are studying individually (rather than learning in face to face groups) and in national or large-scale assessments. The development of computer-based technologies has opened

How to Assess Doctors and Health Professionals, First Edition. Mike Davis, Judy McKimm, and Kirsty Forrest.
© 2013 Blackwell Publishing Ltd. Published 2013 by Blackwell Publishing Ltd.

up many opportunities for improving assessments, examinations and test delivery that were previously unavailable in standard pen and paper tests.

Thomas Oakland [1] describes the impact that computer technology and the Internet have had on assessments:

> Computer use is shaping the ways tests are constructed, normed, validated, administered, and scored. The reach of this technology on test practices is broad and international.

Benefits and uses of technology in assessment

The Joint Information Systems Committee (JISC) is the UK's expert group on providing information and researching into digital technologies for higher education and research. JISC projects and reports have highlighted that technology can enhance learning and assessment in the following areas:

- Dialogue and communication: Online interactions using blogs, wikis, forums, twitter, email and voice boards can enrich feedback and overcome time and distance constraints.
- Immediacy and contingency: Interactive online tests and handheld devices (such as voting devices and internet enabled mobile phones) can support rapid formative feedback, correct misconceptions and guide further learning.

  You may have experienced the use of audience response pads or clickers at meetings or conferences. Often they start with demographic questions such as age or stage in your career but then go onto factual questions or opinion seeking questions. This is very similar to asking people to put up hands. However there are obvious advantages of instant number counts and basic statistics, anonymity (to some extent) with more of a willingness to participate as people can see the results of everyone's engagement in real time.

- Authenticity: Online simulations and video technologies can support risk-free rehearsal of real world skills. These simulations can be done in real time, for example with emergency or crisis management scenarios.
- Speed and ease of processing: Assessment delivery and management systems can provide instant feedback to learners and practitioners, and data can be easily transferred between institutions.
- Self-evaluative, self-regulated learning: Activities such as peer assessment, collection of evidence and reflections in e-portfolios and blogs helps ownership of learning and promote higher order

thinking skills, in turn improving performance in summative assessment.

- Additionality: Technology can make possible the assessment of skills and processes that were previously difficult to measure, including the dynamic processes involved in learning. Technology can also add a personal quality to feedback, even in large-group contexts, and, through efficiencies gained from asynchronous communication and automated marking, can enable practitioners to make more productive use of their time. [2]

The use of technology in assessments can be divided into distinct clear areas:

1. Delivery of examinations and course-based assessment and feedback; computer based testing
2. Administration of assessments, assessment management

Since the 1960s, innovation has occurred in both of these areas to assist in the delivery and administration of both formative and summative assessments in medicine [3].

Computer-based testing

With the advent of the personal computer, computer-delivered versions of paper and pencil tests were introduced. However, these did little more than deliver the same tests through an electronic medium [4]. Now, expanded computer capability offers a large amount of innovation to take place within this new medium. The innovations can be divided into two main areas: content and delivery.

Content

Advances in content have primarily been through the use of multimedia (primarily audio and video) to extend and enhance the authenticity of material used in assessments. It is clear that sound can open up new avenues that could only previously be tested in a practical setting; for example, playing a clip of heart sounds heard via auscultation and asking the candidate to identify the sounds.

The potential of video clips is much greater, enabling the testing of visual aspects such as movement disorders or diagnostic imagery (such as ultrasound or echocardiography) which can be viewed in real time. The combination of these media allows far greater possibilities including whole consultations to be played, following which candidates might be required to make observations, including diagnosis and management, as part of an assessment. These types of assessment are increasingly used in both undergraduate and postgraduate settings, such as Royal College examinations in child health, where ensuring a consistent, standardised encounter with a real child and family can be very difficult.

Computer-based simulations have been developed to cover surgical procedures and virtual ward environments, all of which are valuable tools for summative and formative assessment [5,6]. These types of scenarios enable the assessment of complex (often non-technical) skills and behaviours, such as a video clip of an ethical or legal scenario, after which learners are questioned by the examiner using a standard script. As technology advances and high quality images become the norm, use of multimedia resources will have huge benefits for assessors including greater fidelity as well as being more reliable and feasible.

Delivery

Delivery of tests has been revolutionised by computer-based technology where adaptive testing methodologies can be utilised to make testing more efficient. The capabilities of computer-based testing (CBT) provide many more options than traditional pen and paper tests. The widespread use of computerised delivery of assessments was introduced by the United States Medical Licensing Examination (USMLE) in 1999 to enhance the possibilities of the assessment and to overcome the problems of running a highly distributed examination [7].

The introduction of formats where labels can be dragged and dropped into the correct place holders in high quality screen images allow greater freedom for test designers and a number of new formats for assessment items have been developed that utilise CBT; these are described in Box 3.1 and Figure 3.1.

Most assessment modalities can be enhanced by using features that can only be found on computers. For example, an MCQ test can include drop down menus that display the answer options relevant to each particular stem. Sorting or ranking questions might allow the candidate to display the answer options in the rank order that they have selected. Candidates can be reminded that they have not answered all items at the end of the test and the questions that remain unanswered can be highlighted before submission allowing large tests to be checked by the candidate more quickly.

In addition to written examinations, computers are increasingly used in other assessments such as OSCEs. Typical stations might involve learners having to engage with a data-handling question, interpretation of test results, image interpretation and physical signs or pathology slides.

The computer-based delivery of all question types has both advantages and disadvantages. The main advantages are in the quality of the images that

> **Box 3.1** Assessment formats that can adapted to be used in computer-based testing (CBT) assessments
>
> **Multiple choice questions**
> Yes/no
> Single best answer
> Extended matching
> Ranking
>
> **Selected question formats**
> Image identification
> Drag and drop labelling (see Figure 3.1)
>
> **Free text**
> Text completion
> Short answer questions
> Key feature questions
> Essay questions

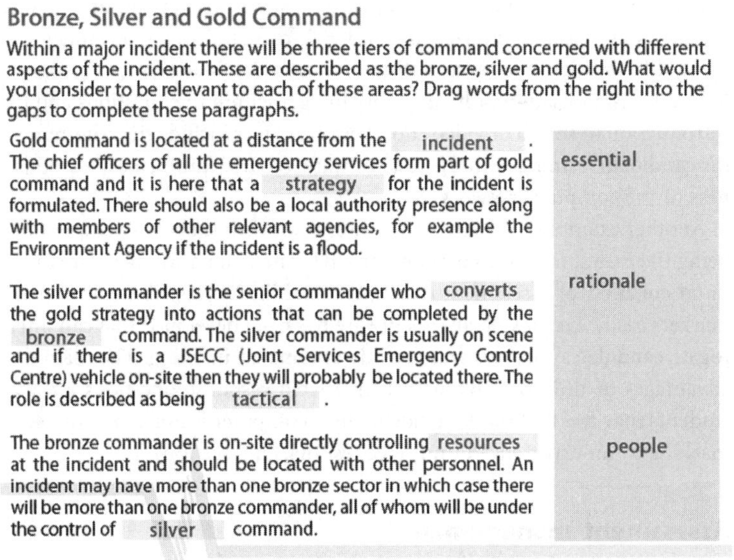

Bronze, Silver and Gold Command

Within a major incident there will be three tiers of command concerned with different aspects of the incident. These are described as the bronze, silver and gold. What would you consider to be relevant to each of these areas? Drag words from the right into the gaps to complete these paragraphs.

Gold command is located at a distance from the   incident   . The chief officers of all the emergency services form part of gold command and it is here that a   strategy   for the incident is formulated. There should also be a local authority presence along with members of other relevant agencies, for example the Environment Agency if the incident is a flood.

essential

The silver commander is the senior commander who   converts   the gold strategy into actions that can be completed by the   bronze   command. The silver commander is usually on scene and if there is a JSECC (Joint Services Emergency Control Centre) vehicle on-site then they will probably be located there. The role is described as being   tactical   .

rationale

The bronze commander is on-site directly controlling resources at the incident and should be located with other personnel. An incident may have more than one bronze sector in which case there will be more than one bronze commander, all of whom will be under the control of   silver   command.

people

Figure 3.1 An example of drag and drop labelling from ALSG MIMMS course. Reproduced from Major Incident Medical Management and Support (MIMMS), 3rd edn, with permission from the Advanced Life Support Group, Copyright © 2012 ALSG.

can be displayed on high resolution screens and in the flexibility of an inter-active medium. The main disadvantage appears to be associated with the difficulty of looking at a screen for long periods, as some examinations can have durations of 3 hours or more, which raises issues with screen size and scrolling through multiple screens. However, most of the disadvantages can be overcome with either advances in screen technology or intuitive naviga-tion options within the examination.

Activity 3.1 How could your past assessment experiences be translated into CBT?

Think of the last exam you took that was a written examination format. This may have been during medical school or your fellowship examination. What are the possible ways that assessment could have been enhanced using CBT?

Virtually all assessment modalities that you will have thought of can be delivered in some way by CBT.

For example, selecting answer test items such as with multiple choice questions are easily converted into a CBT format. Specific advantages to using this are high fidelity recording of a candidate's assessment responses to questions, utilisation of high quality images within the questions and the introduction of sound or video clips. Disadvantages include the requirement for candidate training with the test software, security problems and robust-ness of the computer network.

Another example is constructed answer tests, with short answer questions being the easiest format to develop for CBT. The main advantages are in the rapid collation of assessment data and the ability to distribute answers to markers easily. Free text analysis software has been developed that can inter-rogate candidates' answers and provide automated marking. The main dis-advantages of utilising CBT with constructed response questions are that students may feel that marking fidelity by a computer is not as acceptable as marking by an experienced tutor (see test marking section).

Assessment management

The development of tailored software packages for test construction and analysis allows for greater efficiency in the automation of many statistical processes. A number of assessment data management software packages will automatically carry out most of the routine assessment tasks from blueprinting to item analysis. The introduction of these easy to use software packages has allowed much faster processing of results, more accuracy and greater analysis of the reliability of proposed assessments [8].

The main issue with these software packages is providing enough item tagging information so that the link between curriculum and the assessment items in the database can be established effectively. This type of software package requires constant attention to ensure that any changes in the curriculum are transferred to the question items in the bank. The future of these packages will almost certainly be in the direction of joint curriculum and assessment management packages that allow curriculum learning outcomes to be mapped against the programme outcomes required by the regulating bodies and the linkage of assessment management software. Many commercial packages are already suggesting that they can offer this facility.

Test analysis

Test analysis has improved significantly with the utilisation of computer technology and statistical analysis software; a level of analysis that was previously incredibly labour intensive is now simply and quickly available. It is now possible to calculate high powered reliability estimations for tests allowing the move forwards from classic test theory to the more elegant generalisability theory, Rasch modelling and item response theory (IRT) [9]. These advances allow greater levels of item analysis and have enabled test setters to be able to construct more robust tests with the possibility of being able to predict the characteristics of the test before the candidates sit it. This type of detailed analysis has guided the principles of test design and helped identify poorly performing tests or items within tests.

Test marking

The utilisation of computer technology has revolutionised the marking process for selected answer tests, as optical marking of MCQ and similar examinations has increased efficiency and fidelity. Technology has improved the fidelity of collating test information as hand marking often led to transcription errors and incorrect information being returned to students. The use of high fidelity optical markers linked directly to computer software packages which collate the assessment information directly into spreadsheets leads to very fast processing times for large item MCQ tests and performance-based assessment marking checklists. However, human factors still need to be managed as small errors in database or spreadsheet construction can have disastrous consequences for the individuals whose marks are returned incorrectly, especially in high stakes, summative examinations.

Several groups have been working to advance the capabilities of computer marking by the development of computer free text marking. The challenges faced here are much more considerable that those involved in marking selected answer format tests. The computer has to be programmed with very robust marking criteria for the question to be answered. Currently, the software picks out key words in the response and matches them to the marking criteria. The e-rater system developed by Educational Testing Services [10] marks constructed responses that correlate well with human scoring. A second system has been produced by Intelligent Assessment Technologies which has been successfully used to score short answer questions of medical knowledge. The main challenges with these systems are with complex answers, spelling errors and understanding the context in which an answer is written.

The latest developments in computer-based delivery of tests are real-time computerised capture of assessment data. Widespread use of small and relatively cheap computers has made it possible to create large assessment centres where candidates complete assessments on a computer, thus reducing the possibility of transcribing errors further. The computerised capture of performance-based assessments allows markers to complete an electronic checklist which transfers data back to a central computer for immediate collation. This technology is currently being evaluated as part of the JISC funded Project STAF at Keele University, UK.

Mobile technologies, smart phones and other handheld devices have been explored with workplace-based assessments [11]. At some UK medical schools all students are issued with an individual i-Pad or i-phone with 'apps' for learning and assessment pre-loaded. Electronic log books of procedures and clinical protocols are commonplace for postgraduate and continuing professional development (CPD) purposes.

In fields other than medicine, the use of mobile technologies has been evaluated for the use in assessments [12]. However, the use of this technology has not yet been exploited to its fullest potential. An advance worth mentioning is the utilisation of the Internet for file sharing, which has made it possible to collect test data from several distributed sites and has speeded up the collation and return of results and feedback to examinees.

Test construction

Computers have facilitated significant advances in test construction through the coupling of large amounts of computing power with large question banks. The first steps in this process were to use computers to select questions randomly from a test bank. Computers can also select questions from defined pools of questions, defined by difficulty or subjects, which lead to tests with a higher level of construction [13].

An increasingly powerful evolution of this concept is the development of adaptive testing; high powered statistical analysis has allowed this to become a reality. Adaptive testing allows a more efficient test to be delivered to candidates using the statistical discipline of IRT [14]. With IRT, a computer can create an assessment tailored to the level of the individual candidate. A significantly large question bank needs to be available which has specific difficulty characteristics at the item level so that tests can be delivered in real-time and which will adapt to the candidates' responses[15,16]. For example, all candidates may be asked the same first (moderately hard) question but, depending on their answers, subsequent questions will differ. This method is very useful in identifying areas of weakness for individual learners and stretching the more able student.

A further advantage of computer-based delivery of tests is that synchronous test taking is possible in geographically diverse locations [7]. This is of importance to large medical schools who test in different centres or licensing or national exams (such as a national undergraduate prescribing examination). However, the electronic delivery of tests has considerable security issues associated with it [17].

An interesting development described at the 2012 OTTOWA conference was the development of a computer-based item generator (IGOR) that allowed the development of a large number of multiple choice questions based on one clinical scenario. A computer program would be given a detailed clinical scenario and would then generate a series of multiple choice questions based on the scenario. The initial time outlay in programming the scenario could be realised by a return of a large number of questions in that specific subject area to be used for subsequent exams.

Enhancing learning and feedback

In addition to using technologies in formal assessments, computer-based technologies have had a huge impact in medical education in enhancing self-directed learning and self-assessment (using virtual patients and online tests), peer learning and assessment (using wikis and blogs) and giving teachers the ability to give real time and more extensive feedback (e.g. using e-portfolios or voting 'clickers').

The inverted classroom
The idea of the 'inverted classroom' in which much of the fact-based learning is delivered via computer-based technology is rapidly becoming

embedded in many areas of higher education. The inverted classroom uses opportunities for group work and whole class discussion to apply knowledge to different scenarios, whereas factual didactic learning is managed through self-directed learning using a range of technologies. As the use of mobile technologies in education (m-learning) becomes more sophisticated and commonplace, students can study anywhere they want at any time, and real time group learning is made more focused and relevant to the real world. Group learning gives opportunity for reflection and feedback; it is assumed that the students will already have learned the requisite factual knowledge.

Technologies such as wikis, blogs, Googledocs© or Dropbox© can also be used to help learners work on group assignments. Team working is a very important skill and using online tools requiring learners to work on a group task can help this. Because these technologies are available online, learners can work remotely and in real time or asynchronously to develop resources and materials which they can then submit as an assignment.

For example, learners could be asked to carry out research into the latest treatment for a condition, a public health issue or provide a summary of policy on a certain aspect of healthcare. Using Dropbox to store the resources gathered and wikis or Googledocs to write the document, they then can co-produce a document plus supporting references for submission. Each student can also write about their own and others' contribution to the final assignment. Because this is a multimedia domain, images, PDFs and weblinks can all be used to support the assignment and make it more interesting. To add another (more discriminatory) angle, the learners can also be asked to evaluate the quality and provenance of the references used. This will help learners remain aware of the downside of working in the digital age as health professionals.

Medical students and foundation doctors are now in an education system that uses computer-assisted technologies as routine in learning, assessment and the provision of feedback. In future, all doctors will be required to keep an e-portfolio as part of preparation for revalidation and appraisal, so being able to use technologies to support your own and others' learning and assessment is vital. Where computer-based technologies are very useful is in the rapid provision of high quality feedback.

E-portfolios

In Chapter 4, we discuss the principles of feedback in enhancing learning, using packages such as BlackBoard©, Moodle© and the e-portfolio which can help learners to reflect on and enhance their learning. Increasingly, a type of e-portfolio is being used in undergraduate medical education so that students can gain feedback on their reflections and professional development.

As software becomes more sophisticated, integrated records are being implemented which bring together all data about students or trainees. The idea is that, 'at a glance', teachers, supervisors and learners can access all information about the learner, including assessment results, clinical placements or rotations, absence, application for future jobs, reflections on practice and supervisor and clinical teacher reports. The ability to work at a distance with learners, having remote online access to all relevant informa-tion, enhances the capacity of the supervisor to give appropriate and helpful feedback and support and thus helps the learner more effectively [18].

Some final thoughts

Computers offer a great deal of potential in assessment. They have greatly increased the possibilities available for test construction when looking at performance data of test items. Developments in post-test statistical analysis have led to advances in the reliability of tests and identified more appropriate ways to deliver more reliable tests. The potential for CBT is in its early phase and much development and innovation will take place in this area in the near future. The potential for simulation-based assessments with virtual patients is a very promising area of current innovation that may provide a significant contribution to the types of assessment available.

The range of software and options available to teachers can feel over-whelming, and learners themselves are the product of the digital age, which can feel challenging. However, many examples and resources are freely avail-able for medical teachers through 'shareware' and open access, 'Creative Commons' and 'Open Commons' resources (see Useful resources at the end of the chapter.

References

1 Oakland T. Introduction. In Bartram D and Hambleton R. *Computer-Based Testing and the Internet*. Chichester: John Wiley and Sons Ltd, 2006, p. 1.

2 Joint Information Systems Committee (JISC), 2010. Available at: www.jisc.ac.uk (accessed 4 October 2012).

3 Cantillon P, Irish B and Sales D. Using computers for assessment in medicine. *BMJ* 2004;**329**:606–9.

4 Thelwall M. Computer-based assessment: a versatile educational tool. *Comput Educ* 2000;**34**:37–49.

5 Perron NJ, Perneger T, Kolly V, Dao MD, Sommer J and Hudelson P. Use of a computer-based simulated consultation tool to assess whether doctors explore

sociocultural factors during patient evaluation. *J Eval Clin Pract* 2009;**15**: 1190–5.

6 Brown R, Rasmussen R, Baldwin I and Wyeth P. Design and implementation of a virtual world training simulation of ICU first hour handover processes. *Aust Crit Care* 2012;**25**:178–87.

7 Dillon GF, Clyman SG, Clauser BE and Margolis MJ. The introduction of computer-based case simulations into the United States medical licensing examination. *Acad Med* 2002;**77**(Suppl):S94–6.

8 Tavakol M and Dennick R. Post-examination interpretation of objective test data: monitoring and improving the quality of high-stakes examinations – a commentary on two AMEE Guides. *Med Teach* 2012;**34**:245–8.

9 Tavakol M and Dennick R. Post-examination interpretation of objective test data: monitoring and improving the quality of high-stakes examinations: AMEE Guide No. 66. *Med Teach* 2012;**34**:161–75.

10 Attali Y and Burstein J. Automated essay scoring with e-rater® V.2. *J Technol Learn Assess* 2006;**4**(3):595–604.

11 Coulby C, Hennessey S, Davies N and Fuller R. The use of mobile technology for work-based assessment: the student experience. *Br J Educ Technol* 2011; **42**:251–65.

12 Chen C. The implementation and evaluation of a mobile self- and peer-assessment system. *Comput Educ* 2010;**55**:229–36.

13 Thelwall M. Computer-based assessment: a versatile educational tool. *Computer Educ* 2000;**34**:37–49.

14 De Champlain AF. A primer on classical test theory and item response theory for assessments in medical education. *Med Educ* 2010;**44**:109–17.

15 Kreiter CD, Ferguson K and Gruppen LD. Evaluating the usefulness of computerized adaptive testing for medical in-course assessment. *Acad Med* 1999;**74**: 1125–8.

16 Downing SM. Item response theory: applications of modern test theory in medical education. *Med Educ* 2003;**37**:739–45.

17 Shepherd E. Delivering computerized assessments safely and securely. *Learn Solution Mag* 20 October 2003.

18 Van Tartwijk J and Driessen EW. Portfolios for assessment and learning: AMEE Guide no. 45. *Med Teach* 2009;**31**:790–801.

Useful resources

JISC e-learning programme. Available at: www.jisc.ac.uk/elearningprogramme (accessed 4 October 2012). Contains ideas from higher education about using e-learning in education, assessment and feedback, including case studies in medical and associated educational disciplines.

MEDEV (School of Medical Sciences Education Department) Subject Centre. Available at: www.medev.ac.uk (accessed 4 October 2012). This site has many open learning resources and ideas for e-learning materials to be used in assessment and feedback.

Chapter 4 **Feedback**

Learning outcomes

By the end of this chapter you will be able to demonstrate an understanding of:
- The principles of effective feedback
- The rationale behind providing specific, regular and constructive feedback
- Incorporating feedback into written and skills-based assessment
- Workplace-based assessment and multi-source feedback

The role of feedback in facilitating learning and developing appropriate competent professional practice is crucial. It has been widely demonstrated that effective timely feedback enhances performance and achievement at all stages of education [1,2]. Van de Ridder *et al.* define feedback as:

> *Specific information about the comparison between a trainee's observed performance and a standard, given with the intent to improve the trainee's performance.* [3]

What is feedback?

Ideally, feedback should be part of the everyday learning experience and a core component of the 'developmental dialogue' between the learner and their teacher or supervisor. Feedback can be a simple corridor conversation between seeing patients:

How to Assess Doctors and Health Professionals, First Edition. Mike Davis, Judy McKimm, and Kirsty Forrest.
© 2013 Blackwell Publishing Ltd. Published 2013 by Blackwell Publishing Ltd.

When you explained the likely effect of Mrs Jones' diagnosis of rheumatoid arthritis on her job as a secretary, it was great how you took real care to acknowledge her worries and concerns and were able to book her an appointment with the occupational therapist there and then.

It can also be much more structured, formal and extensive, such as a debrief from a simulation exercise, Objective Structured Clinical Examination (OSCE) performance or workplace-based assessment or a performance appraisal. Most often, especially in the clinical practice setting, it is something in between. Although feedback is often associated with formal assessments and with negative or stressful experiences, a range of opportunities for giving, seeking and receiving constructive and helpful feedback exist on a day to day basis.

My experience of feedback during my training was non-existent. The philosophy was definitely no news was good news! If you were asked to meet to discuss a case or patient, it was usually a bad sign. Thinking back to the reasons for the discussion they were usually around the non-technical skills and the information the supervisor was acting on was from someone else who had told them! (KF)

However, many learners report that they rarely receive feedback and, when they do, it is not timely and, when feedback does happen, it may not be described as such or may not be taken on board [2]. This poses challenges for teachers and supervisors as well as for learners.

Activity 4.1 Feedback

Think of the last time you received feedback on performance (this might be formal or informal).
   What was good about the feedback and why?
   What was unhelpful or discouraging and why?
   What impact do you think the feedback had on your learning or your practice?
   How would you have liked the feedback to have been framed in order to improve your learning?

Your reflections may have revealed that good feedback helps to motivate you to do better or learn more, if it is specific and well timed and it focuses on behaviours that you can change. If your example of recent feedback was from a 360 degree appraisal, it may have included general statements such as '*good to work with*' or '*that could have been a bit better*' which is not very helpful in enabling you to improve performance or change behaviours. Receiving no feedback at all can be more undermining to a learner than receiving badly given, 'negative' feedback.

Principles of effective feedback

Whatever the form of assessment, research (and teachers' and learners' subjective accounts of experience) has shown that feedback is more effective if some basic principles are followed [4,5].

Feedback must be authentic if it is to be helpful and not to undermine the relationship between teacher and learners, particularly if done in a semi-public environment, like a simulation suite.

Feedback must be timely (the sooner, the better) – for written assignments (such as essays or project reports) up to 3 weeks is acceptable, computer marked assessment can provide almost immediate feedback, whereas for practical assessments, especially in the workplace or simulated environment, feedback should be given during the event or as soon as possible after it.

Feedback must relate to behaviours that can be changed, not to personality traits. This does not mean there are no go areas. For example, you may believe the person you have been observing is very abrupt with patients and you may see this as a personality issue. What you could mention is '*You interrupted the patient, for example when they were explaining about . . .*', that is, give a specific behavioural example that you observed.

Try to stay in the present, be specific and give examples and do not bring up old behaviours or mistakes unless this relates to a pattern of behaviours that can be changed. It is essential to suggest alternative behaviours when giving 'negative' feedback. '*Have you thought about . . .?*'

Feedback needs to be personal and individual, related to individual students' goals, achievements and situation. Global feedback can be helpful but reduces the sense of ownership that students feel about the feedback they receive.

Feedback must be owned by the giver who must be sensitive to the impact of the message, but not so sensitive that the message is lost. Consider the content of the message, the process of giving feedback and the congruence between verbal and non-verbal messages. Aim to encourage reflection through open questions such as:

- Did it go as planned – if not, why not?
- If you were doing it again, what would you do the same next time and what would you do differently . . . why?

- How did you feel during the procedure . . . how would you feel about doing it again?
- How do you think the patient felt . . . what makes you think that?
- What did you learn from this session? [4]

Feedback must be clear and able to be understood, whether written or verbal. Think about the way you phrase feedback so that it is absolutely clear to the learner what you mean.

Feedback needs to encourage learning and maintain learners' enthusiasm; it therefore needs to be empowering, even if critical. The providers of feedback are in a more powerful position than the recipients. Gender, culture, ethnicity, organisational or professional position can all impact on the way that feedback is perceived and received and in some cases can make feedback sessions strained and demotivating. Care needs to be taken that feedback is developmental and that we do not use words such as 'weak' or 'poor' (or even 'excellent') as general descriptors, but instead relate these words to specific items in the assessment with suggestions for improvement.

Although giving little or no feedback is unhelpful to learners, we also must take care that feedback is manageable both for the teacher and the learner. Giving too much feedback can be overwhelming, especially verbal feedback. Feedback should be structured and contain manageable 'chunks' of information. For short feedback sessions, a chronological statement of your observations can be useful, replaying what you observed as it happened. This model can be too detailed for longer sessions. The 'feedback sandwich' is a helpful model in which your feedback starts and ends with positive feedback, with the aspects for improvement 'sandwiched' in the middle. Just take care the aspects for improvement are not lost in all the positive statements. It is important not to overload the learner, be clear about what you are giving feedback on and link this to the learner's professional development and programme outcomes. A feedback session should end by summarising two or three key 'take home' messages.

Where your feedback includes areas for improvement you do have to develop an action plan with the learner on how to address this.

Feedback and reflective practice

Feedback is instrumental in helping to develop reflective practice. Kolb [6] suggests that learning happens in an iterative fashion through the four stages of the learning cycle:

1. Concrete experience
2. Reflective observation

3. Abstract conceptualisation
4. Active experimentation

Although the stages can occur in any order in the learning process, feedback is important in all of them to help learners develop and form ideas, get the most from practical experiences, reflect in a structured way about their experiences and test out new ideas, skills or behaviours.

As we discuss in more detail in Chapter 6, reflection can be described in three ways:

1. *Reflection on action.* The learner looks back on a particular event or task and evaluates current skills, competencies, knowledge and professional practice in the light of the reflection, for example in a written portfolio [7]
2. *Reflection in action.* This process takes place during the task or event and helps the learner improve their performance by adjusting what they do there and then, this can be most obvious in the clinical setting where an action's response can be seen immediately in the patient's vital signs [7]
3. *Reflection for action.* Reflecting on and learning from previous activities to inform the planning for the next, again in a written portfolio, but taking what was learned and applying to a new situation [8]

One of the teacher's main aims is use feedback to encourage learners to become effective reflective practitioners through developmental dialogue and structured approaches.

Among barriers to reflection includes a fear of upsetting the learner or of doing more harm than good; the learning being defensive or resistant when receiving criticism; feedback being too generalised and not giving guidance on how to rectify behaviours [9].

Activity 4.2

What are some of the challenges or barriers you have encountered in giving (or receiving) effective feedback?

List these, and some strategies that you have found useful in overcoming challenges.

Providing feedback: challenges

Sargeant and Mann [2] identify a number of challenges in addressing the gap between giving and receiving feedback, listed in Box 4.1.

Box 4.1 Challenges in giving and receiving feedback

1. Teachers and supervisors are often unaware of the positive influence of feedback on learning and performance
2. Constructive or corrective feedback can be perceived as 'negative' which leads to feedback being seen as a negative experience
3. Giving constructive or corrective feedback may be seen as potentially damaging to the teacher–learner relationship
4. Many teachers feel they lack the skills in giving feedback and in dealing with learners who need support after receiving negative feedback
5. Finding time to give constructive feedback is often difficult, especially in busy environments or where the culture does not promote and value feedback and performance improvement
6. Receiving feedback can be difficult, especially when it seems negative, badly timed, non-specific, insufficient or conflicts with self-perception
7. Feedback from someone who the learner does not see as credible may not be well received
8. Feedback that is about the self is less useful than feedback on task performance – critical feedback on self can elicit an emotional response that interferes with accepting the feedback

---

Being aware of challenges and barriers helps both teachers and learners become more effective providers and receivers of feedback. Strategies that help overcome the eight challenges Sargeant and Mann identify include the following:

1. Teachers role modelling the behaviours that they are trying to develop in their learners and putting strategies in place for feedback to be integrated into all learning, assessment and evaluation processes.
2. Combining positive and 'negative' feedback into a professional 'conversation' so that corrective feedback is seen as helpful and not punitive.
3. Taking some time to develop a sound working relationship and learning environment in which the teacher and learner both feel comfortable with all types of feedback. Developing a culture where feedback is actively sought and freely given on a regular (ideally daily basis). Setting realistic goals for learners so they can achieve and make improvements.
4. Practise giving feedback, go on a workshop or course where you can get feedback on giving feedback or ask learners or colleagues how you can improve. Make time to provide support from you or others to support learners who need to improve.

5. Build informal feedback into everyday conversation as you work along-side your student or trainee ('in the moment' feedback). Set times for formal feedback sessions so that this is protected and compartmentalised. Change the culture, starting with your own practise and role modelling.

6. It is hoped that you will not give or receive feedback like this! If you do receive poor feedback, then tell the giver how you feel and aim to have a conversation about the feedback around specific examples or behaviours.

7. All feedback can be valuable, whoever is giving it. But think of the feedback you are giving and in what context, starting small and building a relationship, so that your feedback is actually useful. It is important to establish and maintain your credibility.

8. Distinguish between task focused feedback and that relating to personality factors or traits. Focus on behaviours that can be changed. Acknowledge but do not engage with emotional responses during feedback sessions. Instead stop the session and deal with the emotional issues. Park the feedback for another time.

Incorporating feedback into assessment

Earlier we saw how feedback needs to be incorporated into what Kolb [6] describes as the learning cycle and we have discussed how feedback needs to be built into the entire teaching and learning process. Although in this book we are focusing on assessment, giving and receiving feedback is important throughout the student learning experience: assessment is not just a summative process for the purposes of end-of-course judgements about a person's capacity. Teachers themselves rely on feedback (e.g. through course evaluation) from learners, colleagues and peers to improve the learning process and thus can model reflective practice in their role as teachers and encourage learners to give feedback.

Opportunities for feedback, therefore, should be built into everyday learning processes as part of formative (developmental) and ipsative (where learners are) assessment in the classroom, laboratory and clinical context. For example, in a small group teaching session, you might encourage learners to give either verbal or written feedback to one another on how they performed on a group task or how they made a presentation. Reaching such a point where constructive feedback can be given and received in a safe way requires attention to group processes, providing learners with the skills of giving and receiving feedback and building a culture where collaboration and feedback is the norm and not the exception. The whole purpose is to develop a group that is both willing and able to enhance one another's performance using feedback. Simple techniques like pausing mid-way or at the end of a teaching session to ask *'How do you think that went?'* or *'What do you think you contributed to the session today?'* can stimulate a developmental dialogue around learning and improvement. As we have said, it is important that you as a teacher can take on more 'negative' as well as positive feedback and that you can manage any emotional aspects that might arise with learners.

Feedback and written assessments

Feedback provided on written assessments is very variable, both in terms of the type of assessment as well as between teachers, organisations and clinical specialities or subject disciplines. Traditionally, many written assessments, particularly examinations, did not provide the learner with any feedback other than a pass or fail and a mark or grade. For examinations, this is still the case in many higher education institutions and although learners might simply want to move on (especially if they have passed an examination) it is questionable how helpful this is as they receive no feedback on where they went wrong or where they got things right.

Practical and cultural barriers exist to providing extensive feedback and model answers to learners on written assessments. Often, an examination is put together from a bank of questions which are recycled round year on year. If the answers are provided, then examiners worry that learners will simply rote learn the questions and answers and not carry out the deep learning that would equip them to demonstrate understanding across a wider knowledge base. However, such issues should not stop teachers from providing feedback on examination or test performance. It is good educational practice to provide feedback to learners on written assessments, whether this is a copy of a marked essay transcript, a printout of marks obtained for a multiple choice exam with an indication of what the right answers should be or a group feedback session where the teacher goes through the examination and points out where learners did well and could have improved and provides materials to address deficiencies in learning.

It should go without saying that learners who have failed an assessment or who are borderline need to have opportunity for a one-to-one discussion on where they have performed badly and where they need to focus their attention in order to do better next time. Where learners have failed high stakes examinations and there are no opportunities for resit, feedback needs to be very sensitive to their position and feelings, but also realistic about future opportunities and what the learner might do next. Learners in this situation need good pastoral care, careers advice or sometimes counselling.

Written assessments that tend to provide the learner with more structured and helpful feedback include longer written assessments such as essays, project reports, dissertations and theses. Typically, written feedback will be given according to the learning outcomes, assessment criteria and mark scheme with a clear indication of where and how students have met the criteria and thus where they have gained or lost marks.

Progress tests

Progress tests have been introduced into a number of medical schools around the world (e.g. at Maastricht and McMaster Universities) [10]. They are administered on multiple occasions to measure progress relative to previous individual test performance [11]. A progress test 'reflects the end objectives of the curriculum and samples knowledge across all disciplines and content areas relevant for the (medical) degree' [10, p. 45]. So, early years learners would not expect to perform very well as they would not know the answers to advanced clinical questions, but one would expect near graduates to do very well across all domains of the test. Progress tests can be useful to provide immediate and consistent feedback to learners throughout the curriculum. Friedman Ben-David [11] suggests that a progress test also:

- Samples core knowledge
- May be administered in parallel test forms once or several times a year
- Does not require students to study for it
- Facilitates reinforcement of already gained knowledge
- Allows students to monitor their learning
- Allows immediate feedback through score profiles

E-assessments

As e-learning and m-learning become more fully embedded into health professionals' curricula at all stages, many opportunities can be provided for giving both formative and summative feedback to learners. E-learning has a great advantage over more conventional written assessments as interactive assessments can be built into a learning process around a topic using simulation, games or text-based activities. Assessments are typically often formative self-assessments, designed to provide immediate helpful feedback on the answers to a range of questions around a specific context or topic (see Chapter 3).

Feedback and skills-based assessments

Skills-based assessments have formative and summative purposes, both in examination format and in the workplace. These assessments assess either specific skills and practical procedures (particularly early in a stage of

training or in the workplace) or a more consolidated approach where learners are expected to integrate a range of skills and knowledge. Integrated
assessments of clinical practice are assessed using oral examinations, OSCEs,
the Objective Structured Long Case Examination Record (OSLER) or short
cases. The main aim of introducing more structured assessments of clinical
competence is to improve reliability and validity over traditional unstruc-
tured long cases. The amount and type of feedback to candidates still varies,
however, between types of assessment, the organisation running the assessment and the specialities involved. With large groups of learners taking high
stakes examinations, it is often impractical to give individual detailed feedback on performance. In some cases (e.g. after an OSCE), candidates are
given group feedback on performance and then each learner is provided with
a summary of their performance on each station relative to others. Students
who fail or who are borderline will often be given more specific, individual
feedback with a view to planning how to improve performance for the next
examination.

As with written assessments, new technologies have also impacted on
the way learners can receive feedback on practical skills. Simulated assessments in which learners perform tasks using mannikins or task trainers can
be very helpful in providing immediate specific feedback on fine motor skills
development (e.g. in surgery) or in managing situations such as cardiac
arrest or other team-based events. Simulations are helpful for learners in that
they can practice in a safe environment and develop both technical and
non-technical skills (e.g. communication, leadership) and receive immediate
feedback on performance and improvements. Simulations typically include
a formal debriefing session at the end of the event which provides feedback
to individuals and the group as well as sometimes providing ongoing feedback during the simulation.

Informal feedback

More informal assessment of practical skills and clinical competence occurs
on an ongoing basis and there are many opportunities for giving feedback
to learners through questioning techniques, planning appropriate learning
activities and building time for discussion in everyday clinical practice.
For example, in an out-patient clinic, this can be as simple as saying to a
learner that you will observe a specific activity while waiting to see a patient
and giving some feedback immediately afterwards as you both see the next
patient. This sort of informal dialogic feedback needs to be positive and
specific to help reinforce desirable behaviours: *'You made sure that Mr Y*

was comfortable and explained clearly what you were going to do before you performed the rectal examination. I felt this helped to reassure him.'

Giving 'negative' feedback in front of others (especially the patient) should be avoided. In the informal context, 'negative' feedback needs to be constructive, specific and non-judgemental, with a question and suggestion for improvement: *'When you examined Mr Y, I noticed him grimacing and was clearly in pain, did you notice this? It is really important to observe and stay in touch with your patient through asking him how things are while you are performing an examination.'* Here the learner has the opportunity to say what they were encountering, perhaps they did not quite know what they were feeling for or were unaware of the pressure of their fingers or depth, perhaps they did not look at the patient's face or ask whether he was OK. Building rapport with the learner and modelling reflective practice by unpacking your own clinical reasoning and decision-making processes as you give feedback helps the learner. *'It can be difficult to perform an examination without giving some pain to the patient in these situations. What about if I perform the rectal examination with the next patient and you observe me and how I interact with the patient, then we can discuss this afterwards before you do the next one?'*

Activity 4.3

Taking either a formal written or a skills-based assessment in which you are involved, think about how feedback is provided to learners.

How does this map on to the principles of assessment set out above?

What improvements could be made to giving feedback to learners and how would these benefit learners?

What practical changes would need to be made to accommodate the improvements and how would these be put in place?

Workplace-based assessments and multi-source feedback

Chapter 8 looks at the range of workplace-based assessments in more depth. Here we focus on specific formal assessments used in the workplace to provide feedback to learners on their performance from different perspectives, known as multi-source feedback (MSF) assessments.

MSF, or 360 degree, appraisal is a widely used instrument which supports professional development in many settings particularly where learners or workers are expected to demonstrate high-level complex skills in working with others and where adherence to a professional code of conduct or set of behaviours is deemed essential. In the USA, Canada and the UK, MSF has been used successfully for many years as part of workplace-based assessment for medical trainees (i.e. to support Records of In-Training Assessment (RITAs)) and for qualified independent practitioners (through appraisal and revalidation) [12–15].

MSF generates '*structured feedback which informs educational planning by building on strengths and identifying areas for development*' [13, p. 77]. Feedback can be gathered through validated assessment questionnaires (such as Sheffield Peer Review Assessment Tool (SPRAT), mini Peer Assessment Tool (mini-PAT) and mini clinical evaluation exercise (mini-CEX)) which are designed to obtain standardised information regarding performance from colleagues (peers), patients and others who come into contact with the doctor or trainee as well as a self-rating from the practitioners themselves.

In some schemes doctors can select their raters, which has now been shown to have an effect on results compared with those where raters are nominated by supervisors [16]. In the UK Foundation Programme, MSF assessments has been described as the tool that has the greatest effect on changing trainees' behaviours when used in a formative manner. However, the use of MSF as a high stakes summative tool for assessment is not recommended as it can alter the quality of the feedback given [17]. Once information has been collated, feedback should ideally be given face to face.

A particular benefit has been shown to be the feedback discussion which enables the doctor or trainee to compare feedback from others with their own self-rating. The feedback session should clearly identify an action plan. MSF is not to be utilised as an isolated tool, but as part of a structured professional development and assessment programme. Although the main focus of MSF is to identify areas for professional development, in some cases these processes might identify individuals engaging in unprofessional behaviour. Here, MSF can be useful to identify specific behaviours or patterns of behaviour for remediation. The action plan would specify further training which may help to modify behaviour. In some extreme cases MSF may provide additional information that may lead to medical practice being curtailed. [12]

Case example: The UK Foundation Programme assessments

In the UK Foundation Programme, a range of assessments methods such as case-based discussion (CBD) and observational methods (including mini-CEX, Direct Observation of Procedural Skills (DOPS) and mini-PAT) have been designed to provide the learner with a number of sequenced assessments which, together, form the basis for an overall judgement on performance. Feedback is also provided to the trainee by their allocated educational supervisor.

In addition to providing evidence on safe and competent performance across a range of contexts, these assessments provide many opportunities for formative development and educational feedback [18]. Feedback should be given by observers to the learner at the end of the observation through an evaluation of the learner's strengths and weaknesses with opportunity for the learner to react to these and self-assess. Then an action plan is developed to enable the learner to address deficiencies, which includes completing the forms used in the mini-CEX, DOPS and CBD [18].

This highly structured process builds in feedback and action planning based on the feedback as a routine part of assessment. All the documentation gathered is put forward into the trainee's portfolio which enables a judgement to be made about how many assessments have been completed, the quality of performance and fitness to practice and progress to the next stage of training.

Formal feedback

In addition to clinical assessments, feedback has an important role in appraisal and performance review. Ongoing feedback should have been carried out and issues addressed as they arise, so formal feedback should not contain any nasty surprises. It is important that both the assessor and the person receiving the formal feedback are prepared for the session and that any requisite forms are completed or documentation provided (such as third party feedback).

Individual feedback sessions

Some basic ground rules for group or individual feedback sessions [4]:
- Be prepared:
  - define the purpose of the session
  - make sufficient time

(Continued)

- ○ collect and review documentation
- ○ ensure that you know the context of the feedback (e.g. programme, learning outcomes/competencies)
- Set the scene:
  - ○ create an appropriate environment
  - ○ clarify how the session will run (purpose, timing, structure, outcomes)
  - ○ clarify and agree people's roles
- During the session:
  - ○ encourage the learner to self-assess performance
  - ○ aim to encourage a professional conversation
  - ○ give examples to support your points
  - ○ explore and agree solutions for poor performance or deficits
- After the session:
  - ○ complete any documentation and ensure all have copies
  - ○ carry out follow-up actions
  - ○ make sure remedial or training opportunities are set in place
  - ○ set a date for the next session if needed

Conclusions

Providing constructive feedback for learners can be challenging but is one of the key skills of the effective teacher or supervisor and provides huge benefits for learners. The contexts within which feedback is given range from simple day to day informal feedback, within written, skills-based and workplace-based assessments and formal appraisals and performance review. Whatever the context, giving effective feedback helps learners improve performance and take responsibility for their own learning and provides a culture where performance improvement is part of everyday practice.

References

1 Hattie J and Timperley H. The power of feedback. *Rev Educ Res* 2007;**77**: 81–112.
2 Sargeant J and Mann K. Feedback in medical education: skills for improving learner performance. In: Cantillon P and Wood D (Eds). *ABC of Learning and Teaching in Medicine*, 2nd edn. Chichester: Wiley-Blackwell, 2010.
3 van de Ridder JMM, Stokking KM, McGaghie WC and ten Cate OTJ. What is feedback in clinical education? *Med Educ* 2008;**42**:189–97.
4 McKimm J. Giving effective feedback. *Br J Hosp Med(Lond)* 2009;**70**:42–5.

5 Race P, Brown B and Smith B. *500 Tips on Assessment*, 2nd edn. Abingdon: Routledge Farmer, 2005.

6 Kolb D. *Experiential Learning: Experience as the Source of Learning and Development*. Englewood-Cliffs, NJ: Prentice Hall, 1984.

7 Schon DA. *The Reflective Practitioner: How Professionals Think in Action*. London: Temple Smith, 1983.

8 Cowan J. *On Becoming an Innovative University Teacher: Reflection in Action*. Buckingham: Society for Research into Higher Education and Open University Press, 1998.

9 Hesketh EA and Laidlaw JM. Developing the teaching instinct: Feedback. *Med Teach* 2002;**24**:245–8.

10 Albanese MA. Problem-based learning. In: Swanwick T (Ed). *Understanding Medical Education: Evidence, Theory and Practice*. Oxford: Wiley-Blackwell/ Association for the Study of Medical Education, 2010, pp. 37–52.

11 Friedman Ben-David M. Principles of assessment. In: Dent JA and Harden RM (Eds). *A Practical Guide for Medical Teachers*, 3rd edn. Churchill Livingstone/ Elsevier Ltd, 2009, pp. 303–10.

12 McKimm J, Byrne A and Davies H. Multisource feedback assessment of medical students' professionalism: who should be involved, when and how? *Int J Clin Skills* 2009;**3**:125–33.

13 Archer J, Norcini J, Southgate L, Heard S, Davies H. Mini-PAT (Peer Assessment Tool): a valid component of a national assessment programme in the UK? *Adv Health Sci Educ Theory Pract* 2008;**13**:181–92.

14 Lockyer J. Multisource feedback in the assessment of physician competencies. *J Contin Educ Health Prof* 2003;**23**:4–12.

15 Norcini JJ. Peer assessment of competence. *Med Educ* 2003;**37**:539–43.

16 Archer J, McGraw M and Davies H. Republished paper: Assuring validity of multisource feedback in a national programme. *J Postgrad Med* 2010;**86**:526–31.

17 Miller A and Archer J. Impact of workplace based assessment on doctors' education and performance: a systematic review. *BMJ* 2010;**341** doi: 10.1136/bmj.c5064

18 Norcini JJ. Workplace assessment. In: Swanwick T (Ed.) *Understanding Medical Education: Evidence, Theory and Practice*, Oxford: Wiley-Blackwell/Association for the Study of Medical Education, 2010, pp. 232–45.

Chapter 5 **Portfolios**

Learning outcomes

By the end of this chapter you will be able to demonstrate an understanding of:
- The different types of portfolio used in healthcare education
- The rationale for using portfolios as assessment tools
- Reflective practice
- How portfolios are constructed and assessed
- E-portfolios

Portfolios are widely used in medical and healthcare assessment at undergraduate and postgraduate levels and to support continuing professional development.

What is a portfolio?

A portfolio is a collection of material (paper-based or electronic) that is used as evidence of achievement of learning outcomes over a period of time. Buckley *et al.* [1] suggest that portfolios can be divided into three types:
1. *Collection:* a repository of documents and other materials
2. *Journal:* a diary or story reflecting the learner's journey
3. *Hybrid:* a combination of a collection and a journal

How to Assess Doctors and Health Professionals, First Edition. Mike Davis, Judy McKimm, and Kirsty Forrest.
© 2013 Blackwell Publishing Ltd. Published 2013 by Blackwell Publishing Ltd.

Portfolios typically include requirements for learners to write reflections on their learning through a commentary or series of short reflective pieces. This differentiates a portfolio from a logbook or other record of achievement. In addition to their use in summative assessment in undergraduate education, portfolios can also be used as part of appraisal schemes and in revalidation as well as a basis for providing ongoing feedback and support. All doctors are required to keep and maintain a portfolio as part of revalidation, and they are increasingly being used to underpin appraisal processes. These may be online (e-) portfolios or a collection of 'evidence' in paper form.

All decisions about a portfolio assignment begin with defining the type of narrative or purpose for the portfolio. One of the key attributes of a portfolio is that it contains a purposeful collection of selected student work that provides evidence of achievements or supports the story that is being told. The evidence is usually linked to a single reflective commentary (the specific details of which are mapped on to the evidence pieces) or a series of shorter reflections on separate pieces of evidence.

Activity 5.1 Portfolio assessment

Based on the descriptions above, what type of portfolio assessment have you used?

If you have not used a portfolio assessment yourself, find out about one that you may be required to use in future or that your students/trainees might be required to use.

List the strengths and disadvantages of the portfolio.

What impact do you think this type of assessment had on your learning or your practice?

How do you think the portfolio might be improved to enhance learning?

Why use portfolios in assessment?

Portfolios have a number of advantages over other forms of assessment, particularly when assessing professional development over time. They can be used for both formative and summative assessment and enable the assessment of learning outcomes in non-technical skills (such as professionalism or leadership) which are not easily assessed by other methods. They can enhance reflection and self-awareness although the quality of this cannot be assumed [1,2]. They can also provide a means of bringing together, in one place, evidence of other educational outcome such as certificates, logbook extracts, assessment records and appraisal records. Portfolios can be used at different stages of a student's or health professional's career and thus provide an ongoing record of professional development and growth.

Effective portfolios drive learning and alignment between training and assessment is vital [3]. They are very learner focused in that they encourage the learner to draw from personal experiences and their individual attributes and understanding – no two portfolio assessments will be the same. Portfolios can improve knowledge and understanding in integrating theory with practice [1,2]. Because they require the learner to collect evidence over a period of time (which may be up to a year or more), portfolios enable teachers to work with students to assess progress towards learning outcomes. This can help facilitate a deeper and more meaningful relationship between learner and teacher in which the learner is gaining and discussing insights into their developing professional practice. Portfolio assessments improve tutor feedback to students [1]. Portfolio assessment that requires learners to engage actively with and reflect on appropriate material to achieve learning outcomes can achieve good constructive alignment between intended learning outcomes, teaching and learning activities and assessment [4].

Reflective practice

One of the cornerstones of portfolio assessment is the emphasis on reflection. Well-designed portfolios stimulate the use of reflective strategies and enable learners to develop a reflective stance on their professional development. As explored in Chapter 4, reflection can be described as:

1. *Reflection on action.* a retrospective activity looking back after any particular event or task, and evaluating current skills, competencies, knowledge and professional practice [5]
2. *Reflection in action.* a more dynamic process which takes place during the task or event, and which helps to improve performance by adjusting what we do [5]
3. *Reflection for action.* reflecting on and learning from previous activities to inform the planning for the next [6]

A reflective commentary can enable learners to develop and apply skills regarding 'reflection on action' and 'reflection for action'. Reflections need to be structured, for example around a model or learning journey. They also need to demonstrate how personal experiences affect and impact on the learner's development, and this needs to be supported by evidence drawn from formal activities (such as appraisal or other records, training events, case histories) as well as from relevant literature. Such triangulation enables reflective practice to remain grounded both in experience and in more objective sources.

An example might be an undergraduate student who is developing a portfolio on their experience of an extended clinical placement in a hospice. The reflection on action might include how working with dying patients and their families has affected the student's understanding of the impact of terminal illness and end of life care on the family and how, as a result, they plan to change their practice (reflection for action). Evidence to support these reflections might come from anonymised annotated patient case notes, a record of an interview with a relative or a copy of a clinical assessment by the lead nurse for that patient. You would also expect the student to support their reflections with evidence from relevant literature, for example how the end of life care strategy is working in practice or by drawing from literature on communication difficulties between carers of terminally ill patients and health professionals and how these might be addressed.

Assessing reflection

If you are assessing reflective assignments for learners it can be difficult to decide what criteria to assess them on.

Sandars [7] provides a grading structure based on the work of Jenny Moon which you may find useful.

Grade A. Experiencing an event has changed, or confirmed, how you experience an event(s). You may wish to change how you respond to similar events in the future. You provide an explanation, including references to other literature, e.g. articles or books

Grade B. Involves judgement: what went well, or less well and why

Grade C. Describing an event: recognising how it affects your feelings, attitudes and beliefs and/or questioning what has been learnt and comparing it with previous experience

Grade D. Describing an event: recognising that something is important but not explaining why

Grade E. Describing an event: repeating the details of an event without offering any interpretation

Grade F. Describing an event: poor description of event

Assessing reflection can be problematic, however, in that it can encourage learners to censor their experiences to meet the assessment criteria. The assessor needs to be alert to any mismatch between claims and behaviour (e.g. increased sensitivity towards patients) and to any other demonstration of inauthenticity. Learners may also censor strong emotional reactions to events in fear of them being criticised or undermined by their revelations. A reflective account that was written only for the writer's eyes could be very different from one that is made available for others to read.

Constructing and assessing portfolios

The way a portfolio is designed and constructed will largely determine the quality of the eventual product. Students often struggle with loose open-ended instructions for portfolios and the most successful have a very clear structure, often with different sections for specific pieces of work and supporting evidence. There is evidence to suggest that student led portfolios can produce more insightful explorations of personal learning goals but to achieve this structure, coaching (in reflection) and assessment are required [3].

Constructing a portfolio

The AMEE Guide to portfolio assessment [8] suggests that evidence included in portfolios is only limited by the designer's creativity (as well as the type of portfolio) and may include:

- Examples of best essays or other pieces of work
- Written reports or research projects
- Samples of evaluation of performance, e.g. tutor reports from clinical attachments, appraisal or clinical assessment records
- Video recordings of interactions with patients or with peers
- Records of practical procedures undertaken (e.g. extracts from logbooks)
- Annotated anomymised patient records
- Letters of recommendation
- CVs or biographies
- Written reflective commentary on the evidence and on professional growth

In addition to their use in undergraduate, postgraduate and continuing health professionals' education, portfolios are also commonly used in education and leadership and management programmes as they provide a vehicle for enabling learners to gather evidence towards assessment over a period of time and encourage reflection on developing practice. The case example in the box provides an example of the use of portfolio assessment (using a 'hybrid' model) in a leadership development programme for junior doctors.

Case example: Portfolio assessment in Leicester University's Postgraduate Certificate in Clinical Leadership and Management

Junior doctors taking the Postgraduate Certificate in Clinical Leadership and Management at Leicester University are required to undertake three assessments throughout the year-long programme: an essay on leadership and management theory applied to their own clinical context; a management report on a health management project they have been involved with; and a portfolio.

The portfolio assessment enables students to demonstrate:

1. Understanding of key leadership theories and concepts applied to practice
2. Time management and organisational skills (as evidence of achievement has to be collected throughout the year)
3. The ability to reflect on their developing leadership and management practice
4. Selected specific programme learning outcomes which in turn relate to the Medical Leadership Competency Framework [9] and masters' level outcomes.

The portfolio is highly structured with specific instructions on what it should contain, including:

- Personal background information: CV, mini-biography
- Personal development plans (at the start, mid-way and at the end of the programme)
- Copies of multi-source and appraisal feedback
- A series of short pieces of work in different forms to meet specific learning outcomes and illustrate thinking about, understanding of and reflection on a range of clinical leadership and management issues:
  - review of a book or article on leadership
  - analysis of how you have worked with [your learning] group
  - write up and discussion of a leadership story
  - analysis of a workplace situation involving effective leadership
  - critical incident analysis where you failed to provide effective leadership
  - reflection on a leadership activity/theory from the course and how this enhanced your understanding of leadership
  - a write up of an interview with one of your peers on 'junior doctor leadership' (schedule to be provided)
- A 3000–4000 word reflective commentary on your development as a leader and an action plan for further professional development
- A total of 10–12 pieces of evidence that support the commentary

All reflective and discussion pieces of work have to be supported and triangulated with evidence from your own experiences, the leadership and management literature and course materials and activities.

Assessing a portfolio

The AMEE guide to portfolio assessment notes that implementation of portfolio assessments incorporates a series of steps:

1. Defining the purpose
2. Determining competences *(or outcomes)* to be assessed
3. Selection of portfolio material
4. Developing a marking system
5. Selection and training of examiners
6. Planning the examination process
7. Student orientation
8. Developing guidelines for decisions
9. Establishing the reliability and validity of evidence
10. Designing evaluation procedures [8]

We have seen above how the first three steps might be implemented.
Defining the purpose of any assessment is crucial so that the assessment
chosen is the most appropriate to enable learners to achieve the defined
learning outcomes or competences. Portfolio assessment material or documentation will vary depending on the context, stage of learning and learning
outcomes. Support for students is vital, through mentoring, supervision,
orientation and clarity of instruction [2]. Similarly, assessors need to be
trained and supported. Portfolios have been shown to be an effective means
of summative assessment, reliable amongst multiple raters, although some
triangulation of contents with other sources is desirable [1,2,7].

More student led portfolios do offer a challenge to the role of the assessor and those responsible for training and guiding them. Assessment criteria
are invariably more generic and assessors have to develop the ability to
read the portfolio as 'qualitative data' rather than responses that fall within
strict parameters. This can be a challenge to reliability, and 'credibility' of
the portfolio and of the assessment process is probably the dominant
criterion.

As with any type of assessment, portfolio assessments have some pitfalls
which need to be avoided. In 2009, two BEME (Best Evidence Medical Education) guides were published based on systematic reviews of literature on
the use of portfolios in undergraduate medical education [1] and postgraduate medical education [2]. The messages from these guides were very similar
in identifying the pitfalls and disadvantages of portfolio assessment and
some strategies for overcoming these (Box 5.1).

Box 5.1 Pitfalls and strategies to overcome them

- Portfolios take time: for learners to put them together and for teachers to provide support and to mark (e-portfolios do not necessarily save time or resources)
- If content and size is not specified, portfolios can become huge and a dumping ground for irrelevant material
- Learners need support, mentoring and coaching to produce good portfolios, particularly when they are new to this type of assessment
- They are much harder to mark objectively than, say an MCQ, because of their individual nature and reflective commentary:
  - reliability, consistency and validity need to be attended to
  - defining clear assessment criteria and mark schemes is vital
  - the use of small groups of assessors and discussion between raters can enhance reliability
  - examiners need training and support to mark and moderate portfolios
- The ownership of evidence can sometimes be in doubt, and an oral assessment or viva can authenticate or validate the content

Activity 5.2 Using the strategies

How do you think the pitfalls and strategies described in Box 5.1 are addressed in the portfolio assessment in which you are involved?

If you are not involved in portfolio assessment find out about a portfolio assessment used by colleagues or students.

Think particularly about:

- Ensuring authenticity
- Reliability
- Validity
- Content definition
- Learner support
- Time and other resources

If you need a reminder about the principles of assessment, look back at Chapter 2.

What changes would you make to the portfolio assessment having thought through these issues?

E-portfolios

As e-learning becomes more widespread, the use of e-portfolios is also increasing. E-portfolios can comprise a collection of materials that are ultimately put on to a CD ROM or other electronic devices or (more typically) include web-based resource managers into which reflections can be written, documents archived and other forms of evidence uploaded. Evidence can therefore include many forms of media including video, voice recordings, slide presentations and scanned documents such as completed appraisal or assessment forms. Practical advantages of e-portfolios are that all users can access these remotely without needing to carry printed materials with them and teachers can access these in real time to assess progress and determine if students are falling behind or need extra support.

Case example: The NHS Foundation stage e-portfolio

In postgraduate medical education, trainees are appraised using the NHS e-portfolio which is used in the Foundation Programmes and physician specialty training. The next section describes the Foundation Year 1 programme's e-portfolio assessment process as a case example, and considers its usefulness, advantages and disadvantages.

Foundation Year 1 is the first part of the Foundation Programme, which all new doctors must complete before being able to practice independently. The NHS e-portfolio is an essential tool in induction, pointing users towards their curriculum, helping structure regular appraisals, and in the annual assessment process.

Assessment stages

The NHS e-portfolio [10] contains the following five assessment stages:
1. *Evidence of achievement of learning outcomes* – for example, work-based assessments and training days can be linked by users to the curriculum; course certificates can be uploaded; personal development plans are included; audit reports, publications, practical procedure logbooks are all incorporated.
2. *Reflection on learning* – there is a section specifically for reflection. However, reflection can be evident in more than one section of the e-portfolio. Evidence of written reflection is very variable among trainees using the e-portfolio, as it is not considered an essential part of the assessment process by trainees and assessors. This might be considered to be a weakness.
3. *Evaluation of evidence* – users' educational supervisors are required to give their own opinion of the self-assessment against the curriculum

goals contained in the e-portfolio. Course certificates have to be confirmed, personal development plans are developed and 'signed off' jointly between user and supervisor. Portfolios are then formally assessed in an annual process. Trainees can fail this assessment if all the required evidence is not present.

4. *Defence of evidence* – excellent portfolios which are corroborated by educational supervisors are unlikely to belong to 'problem doctors'. The annual assessment process looks at all portfolios but focuses on borderline or failing trainees (based on their initial portfolio assessment) in face-to-face meetings. In this way, the issues behind the poor portfolio can be teased out, and a plan to remedy the problems formulated. In our experience, a small number of trainees simply do not complete their portfolio in time, and gain the required minimum number of work-based assessments and other aspects of their portfolio at the last minute. This usually reflects on their attitude to learning, and their professionalism, but the face-to-face meeting can discover whether this is the case.

5. *Assessment decision* – the e-portfolio contains spaces for clinical and educational supervisor reports, as well as the decision of the annual assessment, which is based on the evidence contained within it.

Advantages of the E-portfolio

The NHS e-portfolio is high in face, content and construct validity, is feasible, familiarises users with their curriculum and drives self-directed learning. It is a useful aid to the appraisal process as it gives structure and content to appraisal meetings and outcomes.

For example, the user's personal development plan is outlined at the start of a post, and this is reviewed in subsequent appraisals. It allows supervisors to see whether trainees are making appropriate progress in gaining the relevant work-based assessments and experience relevant to their curriculum, and to remedy this if needed. Most of the evidence contained within the portfolio can be checked as authentic (e.g. course certificates).

How users approach their portfolio can give valuable insights in to their attitude towards learning and their professionalism.

Disadvantages of the E-portfolio

Although anecdotally, experience might indicate that the best trainees have the best portfolios, there is no evidence that this is the case. Can trainees simply be good at 'playing the game' but still have problems with their performance in the workplace? What about plagiarism? How *reliable* are portfolios?

In busy jobs which are often demanding, tiring and emotionally draining, the time it takes to complete a good portfolio is a deterrent even to the best of trainees. Not many people are prepared to spend a few hours each month on keeping their portfolio up-to-date, or engaging in formal reflection – particularly if that aspect of the portfolio is not essential to a pass or fail in the annual assessment. The answer to this is that every trainee in the Foundation Programme has an assessment profile.

Assessment profile

An assessment profile (rather than any one single means of assessment) is required to determine whether the performance of a trainee is satisfactory or not. Profiling relies on the triangulation of work-based assessment evidence [11] followed by an expert judgement based on it. The expert judgement lies, in the first instance, with the educational supervisor. This 'global' judgement is important, and in other forms of assessment has been shown to be accurate (Fuller R. Personal communication. The global assessment score closely correlates with student performance in final year OSCE stations. Leeds University, 2008).

The evidence in most assessment programmes contains both quantitative and qualitative information. Portfolio assessment is an increasingly important part of this, but a portfolio is only as good as its parts.

The following criteria identify a clearly satisfactory trainee:
• Timely submission of all the required work-based assessments, with appropriate sampling across the required clinical content as well as assessors
• Evidence of remediation of any earlier identified development needs
• No concerns in relation to probity or fraud [12]

The following criteria each individually constitute unsatisfactory performance:
• Failure to participate in a work-based assessment (other than when prevented from doing so by the nature of the post, ill health or other approved leave)
• Failure to reach the expected standard for their stage of training for all the required work-based assessments
• Failure to remediate developmental needs despite an agreed and appropriately supported action plan
• Any evidence of fraud

Further assessments can be used to increase the confidence interval in quantitative assessments, or to evaluate certain aspects of performance, which have been identified as a potential problem, in more detail.

A note of reservation

A portfolio, complete with reflective accounts of experience, can be an extremely rich source of insight into a learner's experience and, as such, can be a valuable assessment tool. However, it assumes that reflection, particularly that which is to be assessed by third parties, is an unproblematic activity.

The challenge of reflection cannot be underemphasised and there is evidence in the literature that significant barriers do exist [13] and that the reflective practitioner needs to be willing to 'unfreeze' [14] if change is to be a likely outcome of the experience.

Adding assessment to the mix can confound the extent to which learners are willing to share their concerns. There is the risk that mandated 'semi-public' reflection will be contaminated by notions of 'approved' knowledge and fake insight. This is something that assessors need to be aware of.

Conclusions

Portfolio assessment is now widespread in all areas of education. As part of an assessment toolkit it is a valuable component when generating an assessment profile. It is high in face, content and construct validity, is feasible, familiarises users with their curriculum and drives self-directed learning. It is also a useful aid to the appraisal process as it gives structure and content to appraisal meetings and outcomes. For portfolio assessment to be of most use, the purpose and structure of the portfolio needs to be carefully defined and transparent to users. The BEME studies [1,2] have identified that more research needs to be carried out on portfolio assessment to assess its impact on student learning.

How users approach their portfolio can give valuable insights into their attitude towards learning, their professionalism and organisational skills and their capacity for engaging in formal reflections. Unlike most forms of assessment, users' progress can be documented over time and the portfolio can be used as a powerful formative tool by identifying areas of strength and further development.

References

1 Buckley S, Coleman J, Davison I, Khan KS, Zamora J, Malick S, *et al.* The educational effects of portfolios on undergraduate student learning: a Best Evidence Medical Education (BEME) systematic review: BEME Guide No. 11. *Med Teach* 2009;**31**:340–55.

2 Tochel C, Haig A, Hesketh A, Gadzow A, Beggs K, Colthart I, *et al.* The effectiveness of portfolios for post-graduate assessment and education: BEME Guide No 12. *Med Teach* 2009;**31**:320–38.

3 Dreissen EW, van Tartwijk J, Vermunt JD and van der Vleuten CPM. Use of portfolios in early undergraduate medical training. *Med Teach* 2003;**25**:14–9.

4 Biggs J and Tang C. *Teaching for Quality Learning at University*, 3rd edn. Maidenhead: Open University Press, McGraw Hill Education, 2007.

5 Schon DA. *The Reflective Practitioner: How professionals think in action.* London: Temple Smith, 1983.

6 Cowan J. *On Becoming an Innovative University Teacher: Reflection in action.* Buckingham: Society for Research into Higher Education and Open University Press, 1998.

7 Sandars J. The use of reflection in medical education: AMEE Guide No. 44. *Med Teach* 2009;**31**:685–95.

8 Friedman B, Davis DM, Harden RM, Howie PW, Ker J and Pippard MJ. Portfolios as a method of student assessment: AMEE Medical Education Guide No. 24. *Med Teach* 2001;**23**:535–51.

9 Academy of Medical Royal Colleges and the NHS Institute for Innovation and Improvement. *Medical Leadership Competency Framework*, 2010. Available at: www.institute.nhs.uk/medicalleadership (accessed 6 October 2012).

10 NHS e-portfolio. Available at: www.nhseportfolios.org (accessed 6 October 2012).

11 Schuwirth LW, Southgate L, Page GG, Paget NS, Lescop JM, Lew SR, *et al.* When enough is enough: a conceptual basis for fair and defensible practice performance assessment. *Med Educ* 2002;**36**:925–30.

12 Archer J. Assessments and appraisal. In: Cooper N and Forrest K (Eds). *Essential Guide to Educational Supervision (in postgraduate medical education)*. Chichester: Wiley-Blackwell, 2009.

13 Boud D and Walker D. Barriers to reflection on experience. In Boud D, *et al.* (Eds). *Using Experience for Learning*. Buckingham: SHRE and Open University Press, 1993.

14 Lewin K. *Field Theory in Social Sciences*. New York: Harper and Row, 1951.

Chapter 6 **Revalidation**

Learning outcomes

By the end of this chapter, you will:
- Be aware of the assessment challenges associated with revalidation, and
- Recognise some of the possible responses to those challenges

By its very nature at the time of writing, revalidation is not a fully known phenomenon. What is known is that it is going to become a feature of the ongoing assessment of doctors; what is less sure are the precise structures that are going to be put in place to ensure its effectiveness.

Origins and definition

For many years, it was taken as axiomatic that doctors would 'do no harm' and the reputation of the medical profession was, by and large, thought of as good. Doctors might make mistakes, and some were less popular than others, but these were exceptions that could be forgiven.

The synopsis of the Bristol Royal Infirmary Inquiry includes the following:

> [The Report] is an account of people who cared greatly about human suffering, and were dedicated and well-motivated. Sadly, some lacked insight and their behaviour was flawed. Many failed to communicate

How to Assess Doctors and Health Professionals, First Edition. Mike Davis, Judy McKimm, and Kirsty Forrest.
© 2013 Blackwell Publishing Ltd. Published 2013 by Blackwell Publishing Ltd.

with each other, and to work together effectively for the interests of
their patients. There was a lack of leadership, and of teamwork. [1]

This was a collective concern, arising from '*a combination of circumstances*
which owed as much to general failings in the NHS at the time than any indi-
vidual failing'. Among its conclusions was the belief that '*There must also be*
a system of independent external surveillance to review patterns of performance
over time and to identify good and failing performance.'

Such a system began to emerge post-Bristol but not before the arrest,
prosecution and guilty verdict against Harold Shipman who was eventually
sentenced on 31 January 2000 for the murder of 15 of his patients.

Revalidation, then, was considered to be one of the mechanisms that
would offer a degree of protection to the public against the inefficient or the
malign. Revalidation is a single process by which doctors have to demonstrate to the General Medical Council (GMC) that they are up to date and
fit to practise and that they are complying with the relevant professional
standards. What follows, therefore, is an exploration of some of the issues as
they are currently understood.

Since autumn 2009 any doctor who wants to practise medicine in the UK
has to be registered with the GMC, and also hold a licence to practise. All
the professional activities that were formerly restricted by law to doctors
registered with the GMC are now restricted to doctors who are licenced.
These activities include prescribing, signing death and cremation certificates,
and holding certain medical posts in the NHS and the independent sector.
Further information about licensing is contained in the GMC publication,
Licensing [2].

Every doctor needs to practise in accordance with the GMC generic standards outlined in this guidance, essentially, to be a 'good doctor':

> *Good doctors make the care of their patients their first concern: they*
> *are competent, keep their knowledge and skills up to date, establish and*
> *maintain good relationships with patients and colleagues, are honest*
> *and trustworthy, and act with integrity.* [3]

Doctors who practice in a specific specialty are on a specialist register and
have to show that they comply with their individual specialty minimum
standards, which have been developed by each medical Royal College or
Faculty. These individual College or Faculty specialty standards can be
mapped back to the standards in the GMC Good Medical Practice.

Thus, over a 5-year period doctors will demonstrate that they comply
with both generic and specialty standards in a single revalidation process
(Figure 6.1).

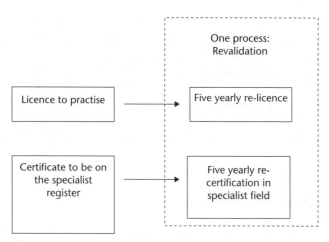

Figure 6.1 Revalidation process.

Aims of revalidation

The Chief Medical Officer of England has identified three main aims of revalidation:

- To confirm that licensed doctors practise in accordance with the GMC's generic standards
- For doctors on the specialist register and GP register, to confirm that they meet the standards appropriate for their specialty
- To identify for further investigation and remediation, poor practice, where local systems are either not robust enough to do this or do not exist. [4]

The objectives in developing revalidation include the following:

- To command the confidence of patients, the public and the profession
- To facilitate improved practice
- To identify those whose practice falls below acceptable standards, and to give advice and monitoring. There should be early warning of potential failure so that remedial action can be taken
- To allow those who are working to the specialty standards to recertify/ revalidate, without undue difficulty or stress
- To ensure equity across any specialty, independent of differing areas of practice, working environments and geographical location
- To be affordable and flexible, and allow further development
- To incorporate, as far as possible, information already being collected in clinical work and use existing tools and standards where available [5]

Essentially, revalidation is designed to ensure patient safety by assessing practitioners in order to confirm that they are fit for practice. This in turn should maintain public trust by identifying doctors who require re-education or re-training. Revalidation and appraisal should allow doctors to reflect on their practice, utilising evidence gathered through practice and audit. Revalidation has updated what being registered means. In fact it is not just about qualification, but also a fitness to practise. Revalidation has also introduced a regular review of any doctor's practice, to ensure that there are no concerns.

The revalidation process

Appraisal

The aim of appraisal is to encourage professional development through continuous education. To be successful, it needs to consider all aspects of the doctor's professional life so that areas of strength and weakness can be identified.

Currently, each doctor undergoes an annual appraisal. However, these appraisals have not been consistent and an enhanced appraisal system is currently being piloted in a number of regions. The appraisal pilots have been developed by the Revalidation Support Team, who have developed a tool kit to collect supporting information. The most recent version of this was published in March 2012 [6].

The Academy of Medical Royal Colleges (AoMRC) recommends currently that any specialist doctor should be appraised by another doctor from the same medical specialty. Where possible the appraiser should also be from the same subspecialty, although it is recognised that in some circumstances, for example small subspecialties or single-handed subspecialty practice, this may not be possible. As revalidation is a single integrated process, the supporting information required by individuals has been simplified. It will be information drawn by doctors from their actual practice(i.e. feedback from patients and colleagues, and from participation in continuing professional develpment (CPD)). This information will then feed into the annual appraisal. The outputs of appraisal will lead to a single recommendation to the GMC from the Responsible Officer (RO), normally every 5 years, about the doctor's suitability for revalidation.

What is a standard?

The following, somewhat legalistic, definition comes from the British Standards Institute:

A definition or statement for evaluating performance and results established by evidence and approved by a recognised body, that provides, for common and repeated use, rules, guidelines or characteristics for activities or their results, aimed at the achievement of the requisite degree of compliance in a given context. [7]

The standard would be consistent across all levels of non-trainee doctor, regardless of specialty. Accordingly, additional standards would have to be applied and these have emerged from the work of individual colleges and faculties who have developed descriptors of the standards required for more specialist performance.

Supporting information and specialty standards

The Revised GMC Framework for Appraisal and Assessment [8] is based on the GMC's document, Good Medical Practice [3]. The Framework has been used by all medical specialties to define the supporting information required for revalidation to demonstrate specialist practice as required by the GMC. The initial standards document set out the Domains, Attributes and Standards recommended by the GMC, each College and Faculty attempted to set Specialty standards against each Attribute. During this exercise it was noticed by a number of Colleges and Faculties that the supporting information was repetitive and an attempt at simplification was in order.

Since the GMC consultation on Revalidation there have been calls for further simplification of the supporting information that is required. All Colleges have developed minimum standards for each specialty which include the following examples.

Generic supporting information

GMC number

Licence to Practice

Description of Indemnity (MDU/MPS)

Registration with the GP

Description of Practice – including title; role; responsibilities and activities throughout the 5 years since last revalidation

Annual Appraisal sign offs

Specialty supporting information

In addition to the specific qualities identified by Colleges and Faculties, there are a number of other sources that may contribute towards an assessment of a doctor's performance.

Feedback

This can come from an number of sources, including colleagues, patients and those responsible for training and supervision. Multi-source or 360 degree feedback has become a feature of doctors' experience and is intended to supplement perceptions from other sources (Figure 6.2).

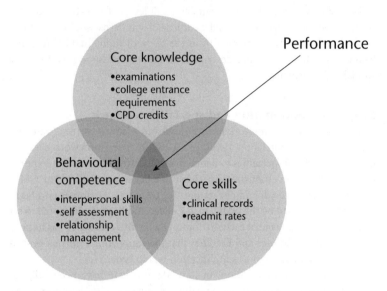

Figure 6.2 Elements that feed into appraisal, based on Dubinksy *et al.* [9].

Some of this can emerge from informal sources, including rating websites like 'ehealth insider'. Launched in 2008, it describes the process as:

> A website . . . that allows patients to rate individual GPs and hospital doctors and share information about their healthcare experiences.

Visitors to the website can rate their doctor using sliding scales for three questions:
- Do you trust this doctor?
- Does this doctor listen?
- Would you recommend this doctor?
  Dr Neil Bacon, founder of www.iWantGreatCare.org, told ehealth insider:

> This is an opportunity to really help improve the care that doctors give. As a clinician, I'm very aware that patients are always looking for recommendations. This site will allow them to see other people's recommendations and make their own, too. [10]

However, feedback is not entirely unproblematic. Evidence seems to suggest that it has formative, rather than summative benefits. Feedback can contribute towards an increased sense of self-awareness: it should be seen as contributory, rather than indicative of capacity or performance.

Other third party information
This might include information on complaint handling (with no patient identifying information), compliments, letters and 'thank you' cards.

Procedural information
Procedural information includes Clinical Governance, audit involvement and management of serious untoward incidents and outcomes (with no patient identifying information).

Clinical outcome data
Clinical outcome data, if applicable, can act as a further proxy for an assessment of a doctor's performance.

Formal assessment
Case-based discussions or reviews or other forms of work-based place assessment (WBPA) and engagement in CPD reveal potentially more qualitative assessments of performance but can be problematic both in terms of procedure and issues of reliability, validity and feasibility.

An aside on CPD. As part of the process of identifying markers of effectiveness in CPD, the GMC and AoMRC came together to commission research undertaken by an informal group from the College of Emergency Medicine and the Royal College of Physicians. The project results were somewhat inconclusive and, in some respects, the final report raises more questions than it answers, leading the original sponsors to revisit the issue in a revised project in 2011. As yet, no results have emerged from this study.

However, the Effectiveness Project did reach some tentative conclusions based on its investigations, which included quantitative and qualitative measures:
- CPD is an essential component of 'doing the job'
- Self-assessment of performance arose from shared CPD experiences
- Perception of peer assessment contributes to self-assessment
- Both self and peer assessment may differ, however, from that made by those with formal quality assurance responsibilities.
- Assessment mechanisms (other than self and peer assessment) are more problematic if they are to be rigorous and robust

- There was a distinction between 'fit to practise' and 'safe to practise'
- Work-based learning is complex and resists easy judgements

This latter point deserves some expansion. Clearly, then, this compounds the challenge for revalidation. While it is possible to 'count' the incidence of CPD (e.g. participation at conferences), it is difficult to assign quality indicators or relate activity in CPD to assessment criteria (Figure 6.3).

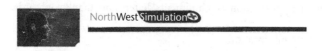

This is to certify that

Mike Davis

attended the annual conference of The North West Region
NHS Simulation Education

this conference has been awarded 5 CPD
points by the Royal College of Anaesthetists

Date: 27th November 2009

Dr Ralph James Mackinnon

Figure 6.3 Continuing professional development (CPD) certificate – evidence of what?

The challenge of all of the above systems is the extent to which they do (or possibly do not) serve as accurate representations of clinical competence (in all of its manifestations). Attempts to clarify this have largely been unsuccessful as medical Royal Colleges and higher education departments have struggled to come up with models that are considered to be sufficiently robust to be confident that the assessment regime is manageable, including from the perspective of patient safety where a patient may be at risk of being treated by suboptimal health professionals.

Among the solutions being explored in the USA is that of simulation. As Levine *et al.* write:

Adoption of simulation technology is quickly gaining momentum for healthcare assessment, licensure, certification, and credentialing. Despite the lack of evidence for improved medical outcomes, the public

*demand for patient safety and growing acceptance by federal agencies,
national accreditation and licensing organizations, state licensing
bodies, educational accreditation bodies, specialty medical boards,
medical schools and local credentialing committees signals the
likelihood that simulation-based assessment will expand.* [11]

The GMC has stated in the Explanatory Note to the Framework that 'No
doctor will be able to provide evidence of compliance with every generic standard.' [8] The type of evidence an individual doctor collects depends on that
individual's job plan, and whether it includes management, teaching or
research.

All Colleges have a Revalidation Committee which has developed detailed
standards and have an understanding of the processes involved. Their purpose is to:

- Guide doctors in their preparation and personal reflection leading up to
  appraisal and revalidation
- Provide guidance for appraisers to discuss and consider the specialist
  practice of the appraisee and to support appraisers in the event that they
  need to explore further any issues or concerns that may arise about an
  individual's practice
- Assist the Responsible Officer in understanding the specialty standards
- Provide support and assistance for those struggling to provide sufficient
  supporting information, for various reasons

The Responsible Officer

This is a new statutory role, the legislation for which came into being in
January 2011. The RO is a licensed senior medical practitioner, probably the
medical director in a Trust or deputy. The role has three key components
described in High Quality of Care for all:

1. *Patient safety*: ensure that doctors are maintaining and raising further
   professional standards
2. *Effectiveness of care*: support professional instincts to improve further the
   effectiveness of clinical care
3. *Patient experience*: ensure that patient's views are integral to the evaluation of a doctor's fitness to practice [12]

The RO is responsible for making a recommendation to the GMC regarding a doctor's fitness to practise and must be provided through robust supporting information presented in appraisal. The standards of this supporting
information are defined in the specialty standards and the generic standards
of Good Medical Practice [3]. For the majority of doctors this will not be a
hurdle, rather a formality.

In some cases where a positive recommendation is not possible, it will be up to the GMC to decide if the doctor needs further training, through remediation or a National Clinical Assessment Service (NCAS) referral, or referral to a GMC Fitness to Practice Panel. This is where most doctors' angst lies as, if a robust and sensible system is not in place, individuals run the risk of falling foul of an inadequate system.

Quality assurance of revalidation

This is an area that is under discussion and there are developments between the Colleges, GMC and other stakeholders. This clearly represents a challenge, the more so the more remote the mechanisms of revalidation are from clinical practice. Clearly, it is likely that there will be varied levels of quality assurance including both internal and external measures. The GMC view includes the following:

16. Day to day quality control will be based on:
     a. Sound organisational revalidation policies and practices which take due account of equality and diversity considerations.
     b. Effective corporate level commitment and oversight.
     c. Robust governance and medical appraisal systems which are capable of collecting and disseminating information to support revalidation.
     d. Effective training and support for medical appraisers and Responsible Officers.
17. All governance systems should be subject to appropriate periodic internal and/or external quality assurance. [3]

This loose guidance does little to suggest the 'who' or 'how' of quality assurance.

Remediation

Inevitably, there will be doctors who do not achieve the standards expected of them. The Department of Health and the Academy of Medical Royal Colleges (AoMRC) are currently drawing up guidance for remediation which will be for any doctor who may require retraining in skills or knowledge, and may involve a behavioural element, involving human factors awareness, which are related to patient safety. This may include a recommendation for National Clinical Assessment Service (NCAS) assessment.

The AoMRC set up a working group in 2008 to consider the relationship between revalidation and remediation and to identify any organisations that might be involved in remediation and any guidance for doctors. In their report they summarised issues affecting doctors' performance including the following:

1. Skills and knowledge problems
2. Behavioural issues including attitude, communication, motivation and leadership problems
3. Working conditions (e.g. team dysfunction, managerial, system or process concerns)
4. Personal problems
5. Probity (e.g. conflict of interest or altering clinical records)
6. Health problems
7. Criminal behaviour

It was thought that most of these would be highlighted in the annual appraisal. The Remediation Work Group has identified the following principles, which should underpin remediation as part of revalidation:

- Remediation is the responsibility of the doctor
- It must be easy to access
- It must be developmental not punitive
- It must be available by self-referral or through mutual agreement with the appraiser, RO, Royal College, Deanery or other relevant body
- It must be focused, discrete and clearly defined (the 'diagnosis', 'prescription' and 'exit strategy' must always be clear)
- It may be intermittent or continuous
- It should be provided locally wherever possible
- It is a process related to, but separate from, revalidation
- It is there in support of the doctor in difficulty with any aspect of performance, appraisal or revalidation

The guiding principles for remediation were laid down by NCAS in the Back on Track Framework [13] supported by the Academy in this document. This group recommended that further information, including resource gaps, was required along with a strategy that would be consistent for all healthcare providers [5].

The Department of Health set up a steering committee in 2010 [14], led by Professor Hugo Mascie-Taylor, to develop the four recommendations put forward by the Remediation group:

1. To establish existing information on remediation
2. Develop detailed guidance on remediation
3. Explore the impact of revalidation on existing remediation programmes
4. Develop monitoring of remediation once revalidation is implemented

Their report, published in March 2011, was based on a set of principles including that patient safety is paramount, any concerns regarding a doctor's practice should be acted upon early and an appropriate authority acts when concerns are raised. Their recommendations were as follows:

1. Performance problems, including clinical competence and capability issues, should normally be managed locally wherever possible
2. Local processes need to be strengthened so as to avoid performance problems wherever possible, and to reduce their severity at the point of identification
3. The capacity of staff within organisations to deal with performance concerns needs to be increased with access to necessary external expertise as required
4. A single organisation is required to advise and, when necessary, to co-ordinate the remediation process and case management so as to improve consistency across the service
5. The medical Royal Colleges are to produce guidance and assessment and specialist input into remediation programmes
6. Postgraduate deaneries and all those involved in training and assessment need to assure their assessment processes so that any problems arising during training are addressed

Essentially, problems should be highlighted early and good local processes developed to support doctors enabling them to accept help willingly. This will require a significant cultural change in some Trusts to minimise the chances of problems escalating.

The group appreciated feedback from employers and doctors that remediation funding needs to be available and equitable, while, at the same time, realised that in the current climate, new funding is unlikely to be available. The group made a number of suggestions regarding this [4]:

• Doctors paying for remediation in part as some doctors do for CPD
• Insurance schemes/loans
• Partial employer funding/link to clinical negligence schemes
• Subscription clubs pooling resources and funding between adjacent Trusts
• Private sector (e.g. locum agencies or industry)

How this report is acted upon remains to be seen but it should be an incentive for all doctors to maintain good clinical practice and have insight into their strengths and weaknesses.

Conclusions

We started this chapter with an exploration of the perceived need for assurance about the quality of doctors' work as represented by some major failings. What we have done is explore the extent to which our assessment models struggle to meet the challenges of reliability, validity, fidelity and feasibility in something as complex as clinical competence. Doctors' clinical practice is enormously complex and is not susceptible to simple analyses and it has become clear that perceived solutions bring their own problems. There is no doubt that this will continue to be a challenge to the community.

References

1 http://www.bristol-inquiry.org.uk/final_report/report/Summary2.htm (accessed 6 October 2012).

2 General Medical Council (GMC). *Licensing.* Available at: http://www.gmc-uk.org/doctors/licensing.asp (accessed 6 October 2012).

3 General Medical Council (GMC). *Good medical practice: good doctors.* Available at: http://www.gmc-uk.org/guidance/good_medical_practice/good_doctors.asp (accessed 6 October 2012).

4 Department of Health. *Trust, Assurance and Safety: the regulation of health professionals in the 21st Century.* London: HM Stationery Office, 2007.

5 Association of Medical Research Charities (AMRC). Remediation and revalidation: report and recommendations from the remediation working group of the AMRC 2008. Available at: http://www.aomrc.org.uk/publications/reports-a-guidance.html (accessed 10 October 2012).

6 National Health Service (NHS). *Revalidation Support Team.* Available at: www.revalidationsupport.nhs.uk (accessed 6 October 2012).

7 BSI British Standards Institute, 2008. Available at: http://www.bsigroup.com/en/Standards-and-Publications/About-standards/What-is-a-standard/ (accessed 10 October 2012).

8 General Medical Council (GMC). *Revalidation: the way ahead* [http://www.gmc-uk.org/static/documents/content/Revalidation_way_ahead_annex1.pdf accessed 20th November 2012].

9 Dubinsky I, Jennings K, Greengarten M and Brans A. 360 degree physician performance assessment. *Healthc Q* 2010;**13**:71–6.

10 ehealth insider. New website lets patients rate doctors. Available at; http://www.ehi.co.uk/news/ehi/3950 (accessed 6 October 2012).

11 Levine A, Schwartz A, Bryson E and DeMaria S Jr. Role of simulation in US physician licensure and certification. *Mount Sinai J Med* 2012;**79**:140–53.

12 Department of Health. *High Quality of Care for all: NHS Next Stage Review Final Report.* Professor the Lord Darzi of Denham KBE, 2008.

13 Back on Track Framework. *NCAS publication*, 2006. Available at: http://www.ncas.nhs.uk/resources/back-on-track-framework/ (accessed 10 October 2012).

14 Department of Health. *Remediation Report: Report of the Steering Group on Remediation.* Department of Health, March 2011., dh_131814.

Chapter 7 **Assessment types: Part 1**

> **Learning outcomes**
>
> By the end of this chapter you will:
> - Be able to recognise the most common assessments of cognitive ability
> - Be aware of the strengths and weaknesses of format, administration and marking arrangements

Learning and assessment go hand in hand in medical education. As senior healthcare professionals, on the one hand we are constantly assessing our medical students and trainees, while on the other we are continually being assessed by our employing organisations and regulators. The focus and types of assessment in each of the above cases is different and so different assessment tools are used.

We might assess students and trainees to quantify their learning and, to a degree, drive their learning. Or the focus of assessment could be enhancing patient safety by ensuring that the doctors who have an acceptable standard of performance are allowed to practise certain procedures unsupervised. The term 'competency-based assessments' is commonly used in this context; we discuss further the assessment of competencies, and the relationship between competence and performance later on in this chapter. Such assessments are linked with career progression.

Senior doctors are also subject to assessment, albeit in a more subtle way. Performance appraisals, revalidation and re-licensing are forms of assessment conducted by employers and regulators. These assessments are also linked with career progression and in some cases the outcomes might influence the privilege to practise medicine (see Chapter 6).

How to Assess Doctors and Health Professionals, First Edition. Mike Davis, Judy McKimm, and Kirsty Forrest.
© 2013 Blackwell Publishing Ltd. Published 2013 by Blackwell Publishing Ltd.

With the above in mind, because the purposes and contexts of assessments vary, so must the tools used for assessment. Taking a simple example of the journey of medical students from year 1 of medical school to graduation, it is clear that the focus of assessment should vary at each stage. In the initial years the focus of assessment is on testing their knowledge and, to a degree, their theoretical application of knowledge in order to solve problems. With increasing clinical exposure, we are more interested in assessing how they can apply their knowledge to clinical situations, in simulated environments in many cases, and then in the workplace. Towards the end of their training we expect them to be able to demonstrate their ability to perform certain skills or to have certain competencies. These skills can be cognitive (e.g. the ability to interpret data and apply them to clinical conditions) or psychomotor (e.g. the ability to perform an examination of the respiratory system). At these latter stages we are also interested in assessing their communication skills, behaviour and professionalism. There is also an increasing focus on the assessment of non-technical skills and attributes such as team working, leadership, resource management and situation awareness.

No single assessment tool is capable of measuring knowledge, application of knowledge, various competencies, overall performance encompassing the technical and non-technical skills and professionalism all at the same time. Unfortunately, what tends to happen is that we start to ignore the areas that are difficult to measure and give these less importance than they deserve. We tend to consider less important but easily measurable attributes and attach high significance to them. A common example of the former is the assessment of overall performance and of the latter is the assessment of knowledge recall in postgraduate speciality examinations.

Charles Handy (quoting Robert McNamara) writes in his book about what commonly came to be known as McNamara's fallacy:

> *The first step is to measure whatever can be easily measured. This is OK as far as it goes.*

> *The second step is to disregard that which can't be easily measured or to give it an arbitrary quantitative value. This is artificial and misleading.*

> *The third step is to presume that what can't be measured easily really isn't important. This is blindness.*

> *The fourth step is to say that what can't be easily measured really doesn't exist. This is suicide.* [1]

Hence, it is important to assess effectively what needs to be assessed. We have deliberately used the word 'effectively' at this stage instead of 'with a high degree of reliability and validity' (see Chapter 2). For the assessment of a practising healthcare professional it is extremely important to understand the factors affecting their overall performance and to use appropriate tools for this purpose.

Classification of assessment tools

A number of assessment tools are available for use in different contexts and for different purposes. Some tools focus on the assessment of knowledge and its theoretical application solely, while others assess performance. Performance is influenced by a host of factors including knowledge and behaviour, as discussed later. A simple classification of the assessment tools is given below.

1. Tests of cognitive abilities
2. Competency-based tests of performance (including work place based assessment)
3. Portfolios

The tests of cognitive abilities are discussed in this chapter. The competency-based tests of performance are discussed in Chapter 8 and Portfolios are covered in Chapter 5.

Tests of cognitive abilities – verbal, written or computer-based

Cognitive abilities can be divided into recall and retention of knowledge at a basic level or higher level of application of knowledge (see Chapter 2) leading to theoretical problem solving, management planning and clinical reasoning [2]. Some tools can be used to assess a range of cognitive abilities while others are more suitable for higher level skills alone (Table 7.1).

The order of assessment tools in the following table does not necessarily correspond with a categorisation of knowledge, skills and attitudes:

Table 7.1 Tools for the assessment of cognitive abilities

Cognitive abilities	Assessment tools
Recall of knowledge	Multiple choice questions (MCQs)
	Essay questions
	Standardised oral examinations (viva voce)
Theoretical application of knowledge – theoretical problem solving, management planning and clinical reasoning	MCQs
	Essay questions
	Standardised oral examinations
	Extended matching questions (EMQs)
	Short answer questions
	Situational judgement tests (SJT)

Multiple choice questions

Application

Multiple choice questions (MCQs) are commonly used in a variety of examinations, both in undergraduate and postgraduate settings. MCQs can be used to test the recall of factual knowledge or theoretical application of knowledge and the theoretical problem solving, management planning and/ or clinical reasoning skills of the candidates.

Format

MCQs usually have a stem or a question followed by a number of items from which the candidates choose the correct response or responses. Questions can be written or constructed in a number of formats. The common types of MCQs are as follows:
1.   True/false type questions
2.   Single best answer (SBA) questions (these can be further sub-classified as)
     a.   A-type: stem and five options
     b.   K-type: stem, four possible options and five combinations of these four options of which only one of the combinations is correct (the key)
     c.   E-type: assertion and reason

True/false type
A typical true/false type question has a stem followed by a number of options, each one of which could be either true or false.

Example of a true/false type question

Pulmonary oedema can be caused by any of the following:

A.	Severe hypotension	T ☐	F ☐
B.	Acute lung injury	T ☐	F ☐
C.	Heart failure	T ☐	F ☐
D.	Smoke inhalation	T ☐	F ☐
E.	Fresh water drowning	T ☐	F ☐

The candidates are asked to choose all, or as many items as they wish, either as true or false. The final mark awarded to the candidate depends on the overall scheme used to mark a set of questions. In the 'negative marking' scheme the candidates are penalised for incorrectly marking items and the number of incorrect responses is deducted from the correct response count when the final mark is awarded. Theoretically, in an exam with 20 stems with five responses each, if a candidate gets 50 correct and 50 incorrect, they would be awarded a score of zero. In such exams candidates choose to select the options that they are sure about and leave the other options blank. In the 'neutral' marking scheme the candidates are not penalised for incorrectly marking items which can encourage guess work. In both varieties the pass mark will be different for the same set of questions and will depend on the standard setting technique used.

A-type

In this type of question, the stem is followed by five options, one of which is correct. The candidates are asked to choose the correct one from a list of distractors.

Example of an A-type MCQ question

Pulmonary oedema can be caused by the following:

A. Severe hypotension ☐

B. Acute lung injury ☐

C. Tricuspid regurgitation ☐

D. Pulmonary stenosis ☐

E. Pleural effusion ☐

These questions could be written to test application of knowledge and clinical reasoning.

Example of an A-type MCQ question

A 70-year-old man presents to the medical admissions unit with shortness of breath of acute onset. His SpO2 reading is 80%, his respiratory rate is 30 breaths per minute, heart rate is 130 per minute and blood pressure reading is 200/130mmHg. He is afebrile. The most probable cause of his acute shortness of breath is:

A. Hypertension ☐

B. Acute lung injury ☐

C. Tricuspid regurgitation ☐

D. Pulmonary stenosis ☐

E. Pleural effusion ☐

K-type

In a typical K-type question the stem is followed by four options and five combinations of these options, only one of which is correct.

Example of a K-type MCQ question

Pulmonary oedema can be caused by the following:

1. Severe hypotension
2. Acute lung injury
3. Pulmonary stenosis
4. Smoke inhalation

    A. 1 and 2 ☐
    B. 1, 2 and 3 ☐
    C. All four of the above ☐
    D. 2 and 4 ☐
    E. 1 and 4 ☐

E-type

These are sometimes called assertion and reason type questions. The first part of the stem is the assertion and the second part is the reason. The candidates are then presented with choices about the validity of these two parts. In this case again there is only one correct answer.

Example of E-type question

Pulmonary oedema is caused by malignant hypertension because increased capillary permeability causes fluid transudation in the lungs:

A. Both assertion and reason are false ☐
B. Both assertion and reason are true and reason is correct cause of insertion ☐
C. Both assertion and reason are true and reason is not the correct cause of insertion ☐
D. The assertion is true but the reason is false ☐
E. The assertion is false but the reason is true ☐

Administration and marking

MCQs test can be administered on paper and the response sheets can be either marked manually or using optical reading devices. These tests can also be administered using computers in testing stations. In this case the marking is done instantaneously and reports can be provided to the candidates at the end of the examination.

Strengths

By removing examiner bias from the marking process, MCQs are an objective way of testing cognitive abilities. The handwriting and presentation skills of the candidates also do not influence the test results. MCQs allow testing of a range of topics in a single examination, making it feasible and cost effective to administer. This format of testing has been used for more than nine decades, helping it to achieve a good level of acceptance by both candidates and examiners.

Limitations

There is a limit to which MCQs can test cognitive abilities. Higher level skills become more difficult to assess using this format, which has to become more complex to accommodate more complex cognitive behaviours. MCQs do not allow assessment of the psychomotor domain. Affective domain can be assessed using MCQs at a very basic level. While affect itself cannot be assessed, the understanding about right or wrong attitudes can be. The MCQ format also allows for educated and random guessing to help in achieving better grades. Like any other assessment tool the validity and reliability of the MCQs depends on the design and quality assurance of the questions.

Essay questions

Application

Although essay questions can be used to test recall of factual knowledge, they should be used to assess the candidates' higher order cognitive skills such as clinical reasoning, critical thinking, evaluation and their ability to compose answers by organising complex information.

Format

Candidates are usually expected to respond to these test items by composing their answers in the form of continuous prose. Answers cannot follow a pattern that can be identified as correct or incorrect against a template. Essay questions are presented to candidates in the form of open ended questions, aligned to the learning outcomes. The questions are posed in a way that tests more than pure factual recall of knowledge.

Examples

Example of an essay question

Describe the possible complications if the National Institute for Clinical Excellence (NICE) guidance for deep venous thrombosis (DVT) prophylaxis is not followed, and how could these complications be managed?

A question on the same topic, but lower down the cognitive hierarchy, could be asked as: *List the NICE guidance for DVT prophylaxis and three ways of managing DVT.* However, this does not constitute a challenging essay type question as most correct answers will fit a template and also the candidates' higher order cognitive skills will not be tested.

Administration and marking

Answers to essay questions can be paper or computer-based but the marking in both cases requires an expert to grade the individual question manually. While it is acknowledged that judgements can be very subjective, trial marking, double blind second marking and group moderation can help guarantee reliable assessments.

Strengths

The capacity of essay questions to test the depth of understanding and cognitive ability is the main strength of this assessment tool. The tests are easy to administer and are still accepted as a valid test of cognitive skills.

Limitations

The number of areas tested per examination is limited by the time it takes to answer a question on one topic. Essay papers, therefore, tend to cover less territory or are much longer than other tests of cognitive ability; for example, the range of MCQs that can be answered in the same time. As correct answers cannot be standardised, grades awarded will be influenced by the examiners' interpretation of marking schemes, whether these be specific (i.e. requiring mention of particular elements) or more general criteria (see, for example, 'Reliability' in Chapter 3). Grades may also be affected by handwriting and presentation skills of the candidates if pen and paper based testing is used. Such exams are also time consuming to mark. All the above factors detract from the reliability of essay examinations.

Standardised oral examinations (viva voce)

Applications

Oral examinations can also test the candidates' knowledge and understanding. These may be used as standalone tests or may follow other modes of testing (e.g. long cases or short cases). Sometimes, Objective Structured Clinical Examination (OSCE) stations also include a couple of oral questions at the end to test certain cognitive skills of the candidates. In other postgraduate and doctoral settings these examinations can be used to test the ability of the candidates to 'own' and defend the work that they have submitted.

Format

In this examination, usually two examiners take turns in asking questions of the candidate. While one examiner asks the questions the other is tasked with marking and the process is repeated. Oral examinations tend to be standardised and structured and every candidate is asked the same set of questions. Despite this, there is invariably some tendency to ask other relevant questions not included in the standardised set.

In the long cases followed by a viva, the candidates are given detailed scenarios, supporting investigations and other relevant information. The candidates spend 10–15 minutes going through this information which is then followed by a structured viva.

In the short cases, the candidates are not provided with information beforehand and the examiners narrate a short clinical scenario to them before asking structured questions.

Example

Example of an oral examination question

You are a registrar in an emergency department. A-16 year-old boy is brought in with evidence of a head injury and a Glasgow Coma Score (GCS) of 6. What are your initial management priorities? Describe in detail your management of this case.

(The initial question might elicit 'ABCDE' (airway, breathing, circulation, etc.) as an answer.)

Administration and marking

Such examinations are conducted in examination centres with private cubicles to minimise distraction and to ensure that the questions are not heard by other candidates awaiting their examination. The marking is done against predefined performance standards and/or criteria. A marking template is essential to ensure the reliability of these exams. The raw scores are not usually used as final results and either pass/fail decisions or percentiles are conveyed to the candidates.

Strengths
Oral examinations allow some degree of free interaction between examiners and candidates. It is possible for the examiners to explore the depth of understanding about a topic using this format.

Limitations
The main limitation is the inability to maintain the reliability of these exams because of examiners' use of non-standardised follow-up questions and overly subjective marking. The variability in marks can be influenced by examiners' own judgement, prior experience and preferences. If in a set of questions one question leads to the other and a candidate gets stuck on the first question, then the examiners would need to provide the correct answer to the candidate before asking the next question. These examinations need to be calibrated to maintain reliability. Calibration takes into account the difficulty of questions and severity of examiners by looking at all ratings awarded to all candidates on all the examination materials. If criterion referencing is not used to decide on passing performance the results are very subjective. They are also time consuming.

Extended matching questions

Applications
Extended matching questions (EMQs) allow more focus than MCQs on the higher cognitive domains of clinical reasoning and application of knowledge, rather than simply pure factual recall. With EMQs the candidates choose one correct response from a list of 8–26 items which makes choice by elimination almost impossible.

Format
Each EMQ has a theme, a lead-in question, a set of 8–26 options and 5–8 clinical vignettes. Candidates can choose an option more than once in response to all vignettes.

Example

Example of an EMQ

Theme: Renal failure

Lead in   The patients below have all presented with renal failure secondary
question: to their medications. Choose the most appropriate cause for each
            patient from the following list. (Each option could be chosen
            once, not at all, or more than once)

Options: a. Chloramphenicol   f. Naproxen
            b. Co-trimoxazole   g. Nystatin
            c. Gentamicin   h. Penicillin
            d. Gold   i. Penicillamine
            e. Lithium   j. Vancomycin

Clinical vignettes:

1. A 58-year-old woman is being treated for Gram-negative sepsis with
   intravenous antibiotics. She has improved clinically but in the last few
   days her renal function has worsened and she complains of hearing loss.

2. A 44-year-old woman with poorly controlled rheumatoid arthritis is
   admitted with peripheral oedema and oliguria. She has recently started
   injections of a new therapy. U&Es: Na^+ 131 mmol/L, K^+ 7.1 mmol/L, urea
   60 mmol/L, Cr 1172 μmol/L.

3. A 28-year-old HIV-positive man is admitted with a 5-day history of
   fever and a dry cough. He is started on treatment for *Pneumocystis carinii*
   pneumonia. Some days later his kidney function deteriorates dramatically
   although his chest infection improves.

Administration and marking

Similar to MCQs, EMQ tests can be administered on paper and the response
sheets can be either marked manually or using optical reading devices. These
tests can also be administered using computers in testing stations. In this
case the marking is done instantaneously and reports can be provided to the
candidates at the end of the examination.

Strengths

These questions are focused on testing problem solving and pattern recognition. There is some evidence in the literature that these questions are more
discriminatory than MCQs.

Limitations
Like MCQs, these questions cannot test practical application of knowledge and performance. Reliability and validity of the test results depends on careful question design. EMQs can be difficult for inexperienced question writers to produce.

Short answer questions

Applications
These are a modification of the essay question and are sometimes called modified essay questions (MEQs). Short answer questions (SAQs) are used to sample a wider range of subject area than essay questions owing to their format. Each question can test application of knowledge, clinical reasoning, management planning and diagnostic skills.

Format
Each SAQ is designed as a clinical vignette followed by a question which can be answered in 10–15 minutes. A typical SAQ-based paper contains 10–12 questions for the candidate to answer in 3 hours. The candidates are required to list, name, explain, describe, discuss or compare in these questions.

Example
A typical SAQ testing application of knowledge and management planning might be as follows:

Example of an SAQ

A child presents to the emergency department with noisy breathing, originating from the upper airway. Please describe the steps you will take in his initial evaluation and immediate management.

As you will see, it is not dissimilar to the viva voce in structure and in the nature of the knowledge being assessed.

A poorly constructed SAQ testing just the recall of knowledge is shown below:

A poor example of an SAQ

List the causes of upper airway obstruction in children.

Administration and marking

These are normally tested using pen and paper-based techniques, but the possibility of computer-based testing also exists. In either case, SAQs need to be marked manually by expert examiners. Marking guidance needs to be developed for each question as some questions may not have entirely right or wrong answers, and in any event, examinees can answer correctly in quite different ways.

Strengths

SAQs can test depth of knowledge and higher cognitive skills. They can also test higher level cognition of ethical and psychological issues. They also allow sampling of a wider area of learning when compared with essay questions.

Limitations

The marking of SAQs is not as objective as MCQs. They are time consuming and require training and expertise. When compared with MCQs these questions sample a narrower range of learning, because of the length of time it takes to answer the questions. Development of robust marking guidance is essential to achieve a degree of reliability.

Situational judgement test

Applications

The situational judgement test (SJT) is a test of aptitude and has completely replaced the 'white space' questions in the Foundation doctor job application process. This test is designed to assess the attributes of Foundation Programme applicants required of the ideal Foundation doctor. The attributes being assessed have been defined by in-job analysis of previous Foundation doctors' posts. SJTs are also used in the undergraduate setting.

Format

The candidates are asked either to rank the questions or to give three correct responses to each question.

Examples

The following examples are taken from the (SJT) website; these and more examples are available in the public domain [3].

Ranking question

1. You are just finishing a busy shift on the acute assessment unit (AAU). Your FY1 colleague who is due to replace you for the evening shift leaves a message with the nurse in charge that she will be 15–30 minutes late. There is only a 30-minute overlap between your timetables to handover to your colleague. You need to leave on time as you have a social engagement to attend with your partner.

Rank in order the following actions in response to this situation (1 = most appropriate; 5 = least appropriate).

A   Make a list of the patients under your care on the AAU, detailing their outstanding issues, leaving this on the doctor's office notice board when your shift ends and then leave at the end of your shift

B   Quickly go around each of the patients on the AAU, leaving an entry in the notes highlighting the major outstanding issues relating to each patient and then leave at the end of your shift

C   Make a list of patients and outstanding investigations to give to your colleague as soon as she arrives

D   Ask your registrar if you can leave a list of your patients and their outstanding issues with him to give to your colleague when she arrives and then leave at the end of your shift

E   Leave a message for your partner explaining that you will be 30 minutes late Select the three best answers.

2. You review a patient on the surgical ward who has had an appendicectomy earlier in the day. You write a prescription for strong painkillers. The staff nurse challenges your decision and refuses to give the medication to the patient.

Choose the *three* most appropriate actions to take in this situation:

A   Instruct the nurse to give the medication to the patient

B   Discuss with the nurse why she disagrees with the prescription

C   Ask a senior colleague for advice

D   Complete a clinical incident form

E   Cancel the prescription on the nurse's advice

F   Arrange to speak to the nurse later to discuss your working relationship

G   Write in the medical notes that the nurse has declined to give the medication

H   Review the case again

Administration and marking

SJTs are taken in the final year of undergraduate medical courses as part of the educational performance measure (EPM) that will allow ranking for foundation posts in the UK. The tests have been introduced nationally in the 2012-13 academic year. They are administered as pen and paper tests by the individual medical schools and marked centrally by the UK Foundation Programme Office.

The SJT consists of 70 questions to be undertaken in 2 hours 20 minutes, under exam conditions. There are two question formats encountered in the SJT:

- Rank five possible responses in the most appropriate order
- Select the three most appropriate responses for the situation

There is no negative marking within the SJT. The predetermined scoring key for ranking questions gives each possible answer a score, based on the ideal answer for that question, out of a maximum of 4 points per rank. The 'select three most appropriate responses' questions allow four marks for each correct response.

The SJT has been designed following review of the tasks undertaken by FY1 doctors previously in post, this ensures that the questions asked are realistic and fair. Nine domains were identified following the review, for inclusion in the SJT:

- Commitment to professionalism
- Coping with pressure
- Effective communication
- Learning and professional development
- Organisation and planning
- Patient focus
- Problem solving and decision making
- Self-awareness and insight
- Working effectively as part of a team

Strengths

White space questions were answered in the applicants' own time and coaching was possible to influence the results. In the case of the SJT the test is taken under examination conditions which gives a better reflection of the candidate's abilities. Ranking questions allow subjectivity to be rewarded when ranking the correct answers. Candidates get zero points for a question only if they put the best option last.

Limitations

SJTs are in their initial phase of development and implementation. Their value in the long-term prediction of performance is as yet unknown.

The responses to these questions may be influenced by cultural differences and preferences of the candidates when taken by international medical graduates.

Conclusions

This chapter summarises the main characteristics of the assessment types for cognitive abilities available to the medical educator. Each one of these has potential strengths and weaknesses and the choice of assessment modality that you make will be chosen to maximise the former and minimise the latter.

Your choice will also be determined by which domain of learning is the dominant focus of your assessment.

References

1 Handy C. *The Empty Raincoat*. London: Random House, 1995, p. 219.
2 Bloom, BS. *Taxonomy of Educational Objectives : The classification of educational goals. Handbook 1: Cognitive domain*. Longman, 1974.
3 *Example SJT – ranking*. Available at: http://www.isfp.org.uk/SJT/WhatIsTheSJT/Pages/ExampleSJT-ranking.aspx (accessed 10 October 2012).

Chapter 8 **Assessment types: Part 2**

> **Learning outcomes**
>
> By the end of this chapter you will:
> - Be able to recognise the most common competency-based tests of performance
> - Be aware of the strengths and weaknesses of their formats, administration and marking arrangements

All the assessment tools described in Chapter 7 assess the knowledge and theoretical ability to apply knowledge in the clinical contexts, which is only one of the many factors affecting performance. The next step is to assess other factors influencing performance which include psychomotor ability, behaviours or attitudes and non-technical skills. These factors should ideally be assessed in the workplace, uninfluenced by the bias of being observed – something which is neither always possible nor practical to do. Hence, we often rely on using assessment tools to assess these factors in simulated environments. Such assessments might have lower validity but high reliability. More importantly, simulated environments offer the ability to alter the emotional and physical state of the candidates and the complexity of the patient's condition to assess how the candidate's performance is affected by these factors.

How to Assess Doctors and Health Professionals, First Edition. Mike Davis, Judy McKimm, and Kirsty Forrest.
© 2013 Blackwell Publishing Ltd. Published 2013 by Blackwell Publishing Ltd.

Competency-based tests of performance

Assessments of performance can be further sub-classified as listed below:
- Competency-based assessments of demonstrated performance in simulated environments
- Competency-based assessments of demonstrated performance in the workplace (work-based assessment (WBA))
- Competency-based assessments of actual performance in the workplace

Performance in clinical environments is a very complex construct and this is influenced by a variety of factors (Figure 8.1).

At this stage it is extremely important to differentiate between *competence* and a *competency*. Competence is a point on the spectrum of performance and it is the ability of an individual to perform a task, while the competency is the task itself. For instance, the ability to perform venepuncture at a certain level of performance is competence, while the task of performing the venepuncture itself is the competency.

A simple model for the competency-based assessment of performance is shown in Figure 8.2. All the tools mentioned in this model are able to assess one or more of the primary or secondary competencies in different environments.

The number of competencies amenable to testing using competency-based assessments of performance can be infinite but some commonly assessed primary and secondary competencies are given below.

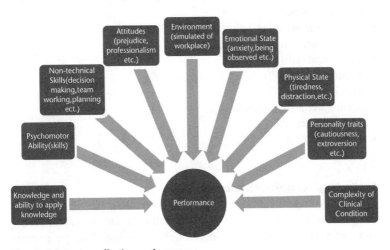

Figure 8.1 Factors affecting performance.

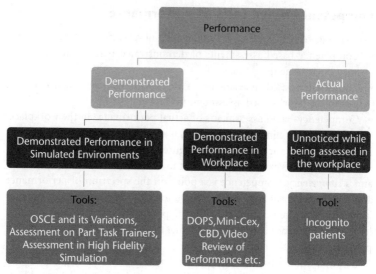

Figure 8.2 Competency-based assessment of performance.

Primary competencies

Complex cognitive, psychomotor and behavioural skills are not amenable to assessment by use of the *tests of cognitive abilities* as described above. These competencies require the use of one or more of the tools available to us to assess performance in:

- Clinical examination skills
- Communication and consultation skills
- Procedural skills
- History taking skills
- Hand-over skills
- Mental status examination skills
- Non-technical skills
- Professionalism

Secondary (cognitive) competencies

These are competencies that may be assessed using pen and paper or computer-based assessment of cognitive skills. In the context of assessment of performance, one or more of these are linked to the primary competencies listed above, hence the assessment tools and marking schemes need to accommodate these alongside the primary competencies.

- Application of knowledge
- Prescription skills
- Data interpretation skills
- Diagnostic skills
- Management planning skills
- Skills required in dealing with ethical dilemmas

Objective Structured Clinical Examinations

Applications
Objective Structured Clinical Examinations (OSCEs) are used to assess most of the primary competencies listed above in combination with any of the secondary competencies.

Format
In OSCEs, the candidates go through a series of time-limited stations in a circuit, for the purposes of assessment of clinical performance in a simulated environment. Each station can either be observed by an examiner or be unwitnessed. Most of the stations include an interaction with a standardised patient (SP). The station duration is between 5 and 10 minutes and the reliability of the whole examination, among other things, depends upon the total duration of testing. Generally, it is accepted that a minimum of 90 minutes of testing, or more than 12 stations, is sufficient to achieve an acceptable reliability (Cronbach's alpha of 0.7).

The terminology varies, for example, the Royal College of Physicians in the UK refers to this format as Practical Assessment of Clinical Examination Skills (PACES) and the Royal College of General Practitioners as Clinical Skills Assessment (CSA). There are also variants of the format of OSCEs such as Team-based OSCEs (TOSCEs), Objective Structured Teaching Evaluations (OSTEs) and Objective Structured Selection Examinations (OSSEs).

Example
A typical OSCE question has the following sections and information in the script.

Example of an OSCE

Question information:
- Subject/topic
- Level of the candidate
- Primary competencies (essential field)
- Secondary competencies (linked to the ones chosen above)
- Station duration

Information for the site organisers:
- Standardised patient (SP) age and sex
- Resources and equipment needed
- Setting up the station

Instructions for candidates (outside the station):
- What is the scenario (briefly)?
- What are the candidates expected to do? (linked with the primary competencies above)
- What are the candidates not expected to do?
- Supplemental data (any further information for candidate)
- Who and where they are (candidates)?
- What has already happened? (e.g. patient seen at the medical admissions unit before coming to the ward)

Information for the examiner:
- Brief background to the scenario
- Examiner's role
- What are the objectives of the station or what is expected of the candidate?
- What information they might be able to provide the candidate
- What information they should not provide the candidate
- Clinical information relevant to the station

Simulated patient information:
- Who they are
- Their social/economic background if applicable
- History
- Details of current health problems and medications if applicable
- Details of their concerns/perceptions
- What they should say (their agenda) and what they should not say
- What they should ask (questions)
- Specific standardisation issues (specific answers to specific questions, please stay with the script)

Marking guidance
- In line with the primary or secondary competencies being assessed in the question and the scoring rubric in use

Administration and marking

OSCEs are often run in examination centres or in clinical wards. It is labour intensive to run OSCEs and needs much organisation. The SPs and the examiners need to be trained in advance. The candidates, SPs and the examiners are briefed on the morning of the examination. Effective systems are put in place to achieve quarantine of the candidates if two groups are being assessed on the same day.

Marking uses checklists with a final score or rating scales with final global ratings, or any combination of these. Each station is marked on the spot and results are collated later. The pass or fail depends upon the standard setting method used. Computerised systems performing final marking analysis are also available.

Strengths

These examinations are standardised and reliable, have reasonable face validity (i.e. they look a little like work-based practice) and strive to be objective. It is possible to have up to 16 stations in one examination and test a range of competencies. Formative OSCEs allow for the provision of feedback to the candidates. The SPs can also be asked to provide feedback to mark the candidates if they are appropriately trained. It is possible to assess non-technical skills in OSCEs as long as appropriate criteria are identified. This is increasingly a component of the work of simulation suites and in more low fidelity life support course simulations.

Limitations

The objectivity built into the system does not equate to reliability. Examiner and SP training are also key factors in overall reliability. Validity of the examination depends on the tasks in question, their accurate simulation and the reliability of the examination.

There is a danger of compartmentalisation of tasks where the candidates do not see whole performance as an important variable and focus on the task in question. These examinations are costly in terms of facilities, time and personnel.

Selection Centre Assessments

Applications

Selection Centre Assessments are an adaptation of the OSCE process, used for the purpose of candidate selection for employment as an adjunct to the interview process. Selection Centre Assessments are now being used for recruitment to speciality training, being considered as a fairer and more objective tool than interview alone.

Format

Tasks may be aimed at the individual or assess one-to-one interaction or team work. How the session runs will be specific to the requirements and the resources of the selection centre. A session will typically run to an OSCE style format, but usually with fewer stations.

Examples

An example of a Selection Centre Assessment

Selection Centre Assessment for GP training currently involves two components:
- A simulation component, consisting of three scenarios:
  - a consultation with a patient
  - a consultation with a relative or carer
  - a consultation with a non-medical colleague
- A written exercise involving prioritisation and ranking of issues and justification of responses

---

Examples of the simulation component can be found at www.gprecruitment.org.uk.

Example of a simulation component

Context:

In this exercise you will be consulted by a patient in an acute hospital setting. The role of the patient will be taken by someone not directly involved in the assessment process, although their written evaluation of your performance may be used for reference during final discussions.

Task:

You have a total of 10 minutes to complete this exercise, which includes your reading time. When you are ready to begin the consultation, please invite the patient to enter the room.

You are a Foundation (F2) doctor working in the accident and emergency department. The nurse in charge asks you to see a patient, Les Milton. Les became very upset while being treated for a knee abrasion sustained in a fall. Les' mother has recently been diagnosed with Huntington's disease. Huntington's disease (previously known as Huntington's chorea) is a disorder of the

---

central nervous system. Huntington's disease is caused by an autosomal dominant gene, which may be identified by a blood test.

Examination of the patient is not necessary. Please assume that any physical examination would not add any further information to that already
provided.

Administration and marking

Criteria for the assessments will be identified based on the role envisaged
for the post, the candidates' likely existing experience and the person speci-
fication. Once the criteria are decided upon, the tasks are developed and
a criterion referenced marking scheme developed based upon the desired
characteristics of the task. This may be a checklist and/or incorporate global
rating scoring. Examiners need to be briefed as to the task, their role and
how to score candidates. Following the assessments it is desirable that feedback should be available for both assessors and candidates.

Strengths

Selection Centre Assessments are particularly useful when assessing apti-
tudes that cannot be easily assessed during the interview process (e.g. assessment of clinical skills or human factor components).

Limitations

Selection Centre Assessments can be expensive and time consuming,
both to set up and run. Asking the assessors to assign a global rating score
to performance can engender assessor bias. The particular tasks need to
be carefully chosen to ensure that adequate differentiation may be made
between the candidates and that appropriate skills are chosen for the individual's level of training.

Assessment on part-task trainers

Applications

Part-task trainers are defined as low mechanical fidelity simulators (e.g.
venepuncture models). These also include resuscitation manikins. The assessments on these models are either performed to assess psychomotor skills in
isolation or protocol-driven life support algorithms.

Format

Such tests can be performed in isolation, for example basic life support
(BLS), or in a series of time limited skills stations (similar to OSCEs) in

simulated environments. The difference of these assessments when compared with OSCEs lies in the complexity of the tasks given to the candidates and an inability to test other related cognitive competencies.

Example

Example of part-task trainers

Examples of tasks given to candidates:
• Perform a lumbar puncture on this model
• Insert a nasogastric tube in this model
• Perform BLS on this manikin

Administration and marking

These can be included in OSCE examinations but ideally should be conducted as separate skills assessments in a circuit of time limited stations. These are usually marked using checklist scoring and an overall pass/fail grade.

Strengths

This approach has the capacity to assess psychomotor skills and algorithm based learning of the candidates with reliability. Relatively inexpensive equipment is needed to run these examinations.

Limitations

These are much more compartmentalised assessments and candidates may focus on the skills aspect without giving more thought to related cognitive domains. This has implications for transfer of learning and competence. Limited examiner training is required to achieve a degree of reliability in this form of testing.

High fidelity simulation

Applications

High fidelity simulation is defined as a technique that involves computer enhanced manikin simulators (CEMS) and the recreation of realistic clinical environments in purpose-built simulation centres or in the workplace (*in vivo* simulation). Assessment using this modality allows testing of non-technical and/or hand-over skills in addition to most of the secondary competencies listed earlier. Although elements of other primary competencies could also be assessed, this very expensive tool should not be used to assess these exclusively.

Format

Each simulation scenario is constructed extremely carefully with a particular focus in mind. The scenarios are run for 15–30 minutes and the performance of individual candidates or a group of candidates is usually video recorded. Typically formative feedback is provided to the candidates in the debriefing sessions after the completion of the scenarios.

Example

A typical simulation scenario can be constructed around the following outcomes.

Example scenarios that may use high fidelity simulation

- Ability to manage a patient with sepsis
- Ability to detect and deal with a medical error
- Ability to work within a team and manage resources effectively

---

Administration and marking

The scenarios can run either in the simulation centres or *in vivo* as mentioned earlier. These are typically video recorded and tagged using bespoke software for simulation. These videos are used for formative feedback or assessment against marking schemes as required. Alternatively, the performance in simulated scenario is marked live by the examiners present on site.

Although marking can be done against simple checklists, specially developed marking schemes encompassing the areas being assessed are preferred. Special marking rubrics have been developed and validated for use with the assessment in high fidelity simulations. One of these specially designed scoring rubrics in common use in anaesthetics is Anaesthetic Non-technical Skills (ANTS) [1].

Strengths

These enable the examination of non-technical skills which are very difficult to assess in the workplace. Scoring rubrics used with assessments in simulation have shown a high degree of reliability and validity [2]. It is possible to simulate scenarios that induce mental stress in the candidates and enable the examiners to assess the performance under the influence of these altered conditions. It is also possible to vary the complexity of the clinical condition in question. These assessments also allow the assessment of the management of acute care scenarios and rare conditions by the candidates.

Limitations

Such assessments are very expensive to conduct. Scoring rubric generation is very specific to each scenario, level of training of candidates and perhaps each institution. Poor performance in simulated environment cannot necessarily be taken as a true representation of performance in the workplace. This lack of generalisability can be a result of limited or no acceptance of simulation as a valid assessment tool by the candidates and the inability to suspend disbelief and immerse in the role play. Such generalisability of the level of performance demonstrated by the candidates to the workplace also depends on the realism with which the scenarios are recreated.

Direct Observation of Procedural Skills

Application

Direct Observation of Procedural Skills (DOPS) is a tool used to assess the procedural skills demonstrated by the candidate in the workplace, in contrast to the skills assessment on part-task trainers in simulated environments. These procedural skills are speciality-specific, especially in the arena of postgraduate medical education. DOPS assessments encompass cognitive elements as well as the psychomotor skills.

Format

These assessments are carried out in the workplace. The candidate chooses appropriate patients upon whom to perform a skill and the examiner observes the encounter and provides feedback to the candidate at the end. The candidates are encouraged to choose a different observer for each DOPS.

Example

Some common procedures for DOPS

- Breast examination
- Setting up an infusion device
- Scrubbing up for a sterile procedure

Administration and marking

The DOPS are performed in the workplace with (importantly) protected time for feedback by the observer. The marking is performed using special DOPS marking sheets. These sheets are modified for each specific DOPS but covers areas such as knowledge, communication, utilisation of resources, professionalism, post-procedure management and safety, in addition to the motor skill being assessed. The time taken for a DOPS assessment depends upon the procedure itself.

Usually, the DOPS marking sheets are included in the candidates' or trainees' portfolios. A specific number of DOPS per semester or year is pre-determined by the regulatory bodies in each speciality to reach a degree of reliability.

Strengths

DOPS enables assessment of demonstrated performance in the workplace. It also allows assessment of competencies related to the technical skill as described above.

Limitations

A certain number of DOPS are required to reach reliability. Assessor and candidate involvement is essential to gain educational benefit from such assessments. The candidates might not choose to include DOPS in which they performed poorly in their portfolios.

Mini-Clinical Evaluation Exercise

Applications

Mini-Clinical Evaluation Exercise (mini-CEX) allows assessment of any of the primary competencies demonstrated by the candidates in the workplace, except procedural skills. The competencies being assessed can be linked with any of the secondary competencies listed earlier.

Format

It is a brief 10–15 minute encounter with a patient that is observed by an assessor who grades and provides feedback at the end. Successive mini-CEX assessments should be observed by different assessors and a range of clinical conditions should be chosen. Variants of this format are adopted by various specialities, such as A-CEX in anaesthetics and I-CEX in intensive care. Despite the variation in name the underlying principles remain the same.

Example

Typical scenarios chosen for mini-CEX

- Physical examination of the knee joint
- History taking from an alcoholic patient
- Examination of the respiratory system

Administration and marking

Mini-CEX is performed in the workplace. It has been shown that between 10 and 14 encounters are required to achieve good reliability [3]. The marking is performed on specially designed sheets looking at the areas being assessed (e.g. professionalism, judgement, history taking and communication). The candidates are asked to include the score sheets in their portfolios.

Strengths

Strong correlation has been shown between the mini-CEX and Clinical Skills Assessment tests in the USA [4]. Mini-CEX also has good discrimination power between junior and senior levels of performance [3].

Limitations

The inter-rater reliability of mini-CEX has not been shown to be very high. There is variation according to the background and grade of the persons marking the encounter. Like DOPS, the candidates are able to select which assessments they would like to include in their portfolios, allowing them to exclude evidence of poor performance.

Case-based discussions

Application

Case-based discussions (CBDs) focus on the professional judgement and previous performance of the candidates in the workplace. These do not depend on observation of the encounter directly; instead the candidates have an opportunity to discuss their performance with the assessors after the event. A variation of this approach, chart stimulated recall, focuses on medical record keeping, clinical assessment, investigations and referrals, treatment, follow-up and future planning, professionalism and overall clinical judgement [3].

Format

The candidates choose a case that they have been managing to discuss with the assessor. It takes 30–45 minutes for a satisfactory CBD, including feedback on the issues discussed. Ideally, this is in a one-to-one meeting in a quiet room.

Example

Any case can be chosen for discussion depending on the speciality and the level of involvement of the candidate in the patient's management.

Administration and marking

This tool can be used in a variety of workplaces including clinics and operating theatres. The number of cases required by the candidate is determined by the educational authorities in their speciality but generally 4–6 cases each year are considered satisfactory. The marking is once again performed on specially designed forms and can focus on any of the areas chosen for assessment described under the application heading above.

Strengths

CBDs have shown good reliability and validity. They allow the assessors to use questioning to probe the reasoning behind decision making and induce metacognition (thinking about the thinking) and reflection.

Limitations

There are limited data on the educational impact of CBDs. Like DOPS and mini-CEX, the candidates have the freedom to choose which reports to include in their portfolios.

Video review of performance

Application

The Royal College of General Practitioners refer to this as Consultation Observation Tool (COT). Essentially, this is similar to mini-CEX but with a *post hoc* video analysis. Its applications are similar to mini-CEX described above.

Format

A prospective consultation is agreed upon by the candidate and the assessor for video recording. The candidates are allowed to make a number of videos and choose one or more to submit for assessment. The video duration would depend upon the nature of the consultation.

Administration and marking

Special consideration in this form of assessment is needed for the consent for video recording of the patients. In the UK, generally patients younger than 10 years and older than 75 years of age or those with mental health problems are not chosen. The marking is done by the examiner in the presence of the candidates against pre-set competency-based criteria.

Strengths

The ability to locate and focus electronically on specific areas is a great strength of this tool. Furthermore, the candidates are able to watch and reflect on their own performance. This enables close attention to data, as opposed to (possibly competing) interpretations of them.

Limitations

It is not possible to video all consultations of educational importance because of the sensitive nature of discussions, privacy and dignity issue or age of the patients.

Incognito patients

Applications

This is the only tool available for the assessment of actual performance. In this type of assessment trained assessors are disguised as patients who have consultations with the candidates and mark their performance. This mode of assessment is able to assess most of the primary and secondary competencies, except procedural skills, with a very high degree of validity.

Format

The candidates are informed that during their clinics there will be one incognito patient on that day or in the next few days. A trained assessor then has a consultation with the candidate and grades their performance. Alternatively, existing patients can be trained to become assessors for this purpose.

Administration and marking

This format of examination is more suitable for outpatient or GP consultations. The examiners need to be properly trained to be able to conceal their identity. There is good evidence that candidates are unable to detect the incognito patient. The marking is done against pre-set criteria.

Strengths

The greatest strength of this assessment tool is its ability to sample actual performance with a high degree of validity.

Limitations

It is difficult to use this technique of assessment in inpatient wards and for procedural skills. If the candidates are able to detect the incognito patient then their performance is biased and true performance is not captured.

Portfolios

The areas assessed by portfolios include assessment of professionalism and reflective practice as discussed in detail in Chapter 6.

Conclusions

This and the previous chapter summarises the main characteristics of the assessment types available to the medical educator. Each assessment type has potential strengths and weaknesses and by choosing the right modality the educator should maximise the former and minimise the latter. The choice will also be determined by which domain of learning is the dominant focus of assessment.

References

1 Fletcher G, Flin R, McGeorge P, Maran N and Patey R. Anaesthetists' Non-Technical Skills (ANTS): evaluation of a behavioural marker system. *Br J Anaesth* 2003; **90**:580–8.

2 Khan K, Tolhurst-Cleaver S, White S and Simpson P. *Simulation in Healthcare Education, building a simulation programme: A practical guide.* Dundee: AMEE, 2011.

3 Boursicot K, Etheridge L, Setna Z, Sturrock A, Ker J, Smee S, et al. Performance in assessment: Consensus statement and recommendations from the Ottawa conference. *Med Teach* 2011;**33**:370–83.

4 Boulet JR, McKinley DW, Norcini JJ and Whelan GP. Assessing the comparability of standardized patient and physician evaluations of clinical skills. *Adv Health Sci Educ Theory Pract* 2002;**7**:85–97.

Chapter 9 **Programmatic assessment**

Learning outcomes

By the end of this chapter, you will:
- Be able to recognise the need for programme assessment
- Be aware of one approach to this

In Chapter 2 we discussed the reasons why we assess. One of the possible answers to the question was to measure the effectiveness of the teaching. Poor results from groups of learners would obviously raise questions about how a programme was being taught. Another reason for assessment which looks at the origins of an assessment regime, rather than its subjects, is the need to look closely at programmes: their structure, presentation and selection of assessment tools. The Royal College that found itself failing all but 2% of its first overseas examinations had to look long and hard at how it assessed rather than simply blaming the students for their ignorance.

In order to choose appropriate assessment tools for the right purposes it is essential to know what is important to assess. This can be done by identifying the learning objectives or outcomes of a teaching programme and then choosing appropriate assessment tools to target these areas. This is known as blueprinting. For example, if the outcomes of a speciality training programme include having knowledge about specific conditions, the ability to perform certain skills, being a good team leader and player, the ability to act professionally and to perform well under stressful situations, then the combination of assessments should be able to target all these areas.

How to Assess Doctors and Health Professionals, First Edition. Mike Davis, Judy McKimm, and Kirsty Forrest.
© 2013 Blackwell Publishing Ltd. Published 2013 by Blackwell Publishing Ltd.

Traditionally, as we explore in Chapter 3, assessment has been classified into formative and summative types. More recently, the literature in medical education is favouring the use of the terms: low, medium and high stakes assessments instead [1]. In the low stakes assessments (formative assessments or assessment for learning), the results do not have direct major consequences on the promotion or career progression of the candidates, while the high stakes assessments would have the same standing as the traditional pass/fail summative assessments. In this spectrum, medium stakes assessments would bear more weight than the low stakes assessments (e.g. semester tests), but have a lesser impact on the candidates' progression in the case of poor performance.

Van der Vleuten *et al.* [1] have described programmatic assessment as a methodology to collect data from low and medium stakes assessments longitudinally and use them to come to high stakes decisions. Each assessment result is considered as a data point and the higher the stakes the more data points are needed for aggregation to come to a decision. It is very important to understand that such aggregation is not quantitative (i.e. it is not summation or averaging of scores), rather it is aggregation and interpretation of rich qualitative, and at other times quantitative, data by experts.

In order to be able to assess a wide range of 'cognitive, affective and psychomotor abilities' and performance in a range of clinical situations, a test battery approach should be employed longitudinally. In such a test battery a combination of assessment tools should be utilised, sampling all the outcomes required of the teaching or training programme. The data should be collected over a period of time (longitudinally) and the results will then depend on the aggregation of results. These results can be aggregated at intermediate points during a programme and/or at the end of the programme [1].

To explain this concept further we would like to use the example of undergraduate medical education outcomes and standards set out in *Tomorrow's Doctors, 2009* (General Medical Council, 2009) and propose an 'ideal' assessment programme which would have been preceded by a 'mapping' of learning outcomes to teaching and learning episodes.

An ideal programmatic assessment for outcomes set in *Tomorrow's Doctors 2009*

In order to propose a programme suitable for the assessment of the outcomes set in *Tomorrow's Doctors, 2009*, it is important to have a brief overview of what is required of medical graduates in the UK. There are 16 high level outcomes set out under three categories:

1. Doctor as scholar and scientist
2. Doctor as professional
3. Doctor as practitioner

In addition, graduates are expected to have acceptable standards of performance on 32 practical skills.

We are using the example of the first broad outcome, 'doctor as scholar and scientist', and a selection of its sub-domains to show how a variety of assessment tools would be needed to assess these outcomes programmatically (Table 9.1).

The selected outcomes are shown in the first column of Table 9.1. The second column shows the proposed assessment tools that could be used to assess these outcomes. The third column shows the stage in a typical 5-year programme at which the assessment should ideally be conducted. This table should be seen as an example rather than a definitive prescription for conducting assessments. There will always be scope for using alternate assessment tools at different points in the programme depending on the mode of delivery of the curriculum.

This way of looking at particular outcomes and aligning these to the assessments used will reveal any inadequacies in a programme. When looking at a whole programme assessment strategy, those responsible for programmes can identify possible assessment regimes that need to be reviewed and improved.

Programme designers must remember:

> a coherent system of assessment crystallizes for learners and the public the priorities and values of those who set it up, and who, as a result, inevitably promote a particular set of educational and professional values. [2]

Table 9.1 Five outcomes under 'The doctor as a scholar and a scientist'

Outcomes	Proposed assessment	Stage (year)
The graduate will be able to apply to medical practice biomedical scientific principles, method and knowledge relating to: anatomy, biochemistry, cell biology, genetics, immunology, microbiology, molecular biology, nutrition, pathology, pharmacology and physiology		
(a) Explain normal human structure and functions	Viva voce, essay type questions	1–2
(b) Explain the scientific bases for common disease presentations	Viva voce, essay type questions	1–2
(c) Justify the selection of appropriate investigations for common clinical cases	Viva voce, essay type questions	3–5
(d) Explain the fundamental principles underlying such investigative techniques	Viva voce, essay type questions	3–5
(e) Select appropriate forms of management for common diseases and ways of preventing common diseases, and explain their modes of action and their risks from first principles	MCQs/EMQs, script concordance tests, viva voce, essay type questions, OSCEs	1–5
(f) Demonstrate knowledge of drug actions: therapeutics and pharmacokinetics; drug side effects and interactions, including for multiple treatments, long-term conditions and non-prescribed medication; and also including effects on the population, such as the spread of antibiotic resistance	MCQs/EMQs, script concordance tests, viva voce, essay type questions, prescription skills assessment	1–5
(g) Make accurate observations of clinical phenomena and appropriate critical analysis of clinical data	CBD, Mini-CEX, OSCE, assessment using computer enhanced manikin simulation (CEMS)	3–5
Apply psychological principles, method and knowledge to medical practice		
(a) Explain normal human behaviour at an individual level	Viva voce, essay type questions	1–5
(b) Discuss psychological concepts of health, illness and disease	Viva voce, essay type questions	1–5
(c) Apply theoretical frameworks of psychology to explain the varied responses of individuals, groups and societies to disease	Viva voce, essay type questions	1–5
(d) Explain psychological factors that contribute to illness, the course of the disease and the success of treatment	Viva voce, essay type questions	1–5

(Continued)

Table 9.1 (*Continued*)

Outcomes	Proposed assessment	Stage (year)
(e) Discuss psychological aspects of behavioural change and treatment compliance	Viva voce, essay type questions	1–5
(f) Discuss adaptation to major life changes, such as bereavement; comparing and contrasting the abnormal adjustments that might occur in these situations	Viva voce, essay type questions	1–5
(g) Identify appropriate strategies for managing patients with dependence issues and other demonstrations of self-harm	Viva voce, essay type questions MCQs/EMQs Script concordance	1–5
Apply social science principles, method and knowledge to medical practice		
(a) Explain normal human behaviour at a societal level	Viva voce, essay type questions	1–5
(b) Discuss sociological concepts of health, illness and disease	Viva voce, essay type questions	1–5
(c) Apply theoretical frameworks of sociology to explain the varied responses of individuals, groups and societies to disease	Viva voce, essay type questions	1–5
(d) Explain sociological factors that contribute to illness, the course of the disease and the success of treatment – including issues relating to health inequalities, the links between occupation and health and the effects of poverty and affluence	Viva voce, essay type questions	1–5
(e) Discuss sociological aspects of behavioural change and treatment compliance	Viva voce, essay type questions	1–5
Apply to medical practice the principles, method and knowledge of population health and the improvement of health and healthcare		
(a) Discuss basic principles of health improvement, including the wider determinants of health, health inequalities, health risks and disease surveillance	Viva voce, essay type questions	1–5
(b) Assess how health behaviours and outcomes are affected by the diversity of the patient population	Viva voce, essay type questions, OSCEs, CBDs	1–5
(c) Describe measurement methods relevant to the improvement of clinical effectiveness and care	Viva voce, essay type questions	1–5

Table 9.1 (*Continued*)

Outcomes	Proposed assessment	Stage (year)
(d) Discuss the principles underlying the development of health and health service policy, including issues relating to health economics and equity, and clinical guidelines	Viva voce, essay type questions	1–5
(e) Explain and apply the basic principles of communicable disease control in hospital and community settings	Viva voce, essay type questions, DOPS, mini-CEX, OSCEs	3–5
(f) Evaluate and apply epidemiological data in managing healthcare for the individual and the community	Viva voce, essay type questions	1–5
(g) Recognise the role of environmental and occupational hazards in ill-health and discuss ways to mitigate their effects	Viva voce, essay type questions	1–5
(h) Discuss the role of nutrition in health	Viva voce, essay type questions, CBDs	1–5
(i) Discuss the principles and application of primary, secondary and tertiary prevention of disease	Viva voce, essay type questions, OSCEs, CBDs	1–5
(j) Discuss from a global perspective the determinants of health and disease and variations in healthcare delivery and medical practice	Viva voce, essay type questions	1–5
Apply scientific method and approaches to medical research		
(a) Critically appraise the results of relevant diagnostic, prognostic and treatment trials and other qualitative and quantitative studies as reported in the medical and scientific literature	Desktop literature review projects	1–5
(b) Formulate simple relevant research questions in biomedical science, psychosocial science or population science, and design appropriate studies or experiments to address the questions	SSCs, projects	1–5
(c) Apply findings from the literature to answer questions raised by specific clinical problems	Essay type questions, CBDs	1–5
(d) Understand the ethical and governance issues involved in medical research	Viva voce, essay type questions, research projects	1–5

This process does not have to be as extensive as looking at the curriculum for a medical school. You can apply these same principles to your own teaching no matter what the scale. Table 9.2 is an example of a workshop delivered to Year 5 medical students about acute care. Thinking of what assessment to use and where it shoud be carried out is important when planning the content of your teaching.

Objectives

By the end of the day the students will:
• Be able to recognise an acutely ill patient
• Initially manage an acutely ill patient
• Communicate effectively to senior colleagues about an acutely ill patient
• Understand the bigger picture regarding acute care in the National Health Service (NHS)

Table 9.2 Example workshop plan: Acute care training for Year 5 medical students

Time	Subject	Assessment
0900–0930	Registration and coffee	Self-assessed MCQ
0930–1030	Lecture: recognising critical illness and the ABCDE system	Included reflection on unwell patients they had observed and cardiac arrests that had not gone well
1030–1115 1115–1200	Split in to two tutorial groups: • Oxygen therapy • Blood gases	Oxygen and blood gas quiz used throughout the workshops
1200–1215	1200–1215 SimMan™ demonstration	
1215–1245	Lunch	
1245–1415 Coffee 1430–1600	Split in to two groups: • Fluids and volume • Simulated scenarios resuscitation using SimMan™	Fluids quiz used throughout workshop. Simulated scenarios – facilitated peer led assessment of performance. Assessment of skills performed on manikin
1600–1620	Short lecture: summary of the ABCDE system	
1620–1630 Few weeks later	Course evaluation	Repeat self-assessed MCQ OSCE designed for the final MBChB exam

Summary

This chapter has looked at an approach to planning and evaluating an assessment programme (through the use of blueprinting and mapping) is designed to encourage users to reflect on the impact of chosen assessment tools and to consider their effectiveness and efficiency.

References

1 Van der Vleuten CP, Schuwirth LW, Driessen EW, Dijkstra J, Tigelaar D, Baartman LK, *et al.* A model for programmatic assessment fit for purpose. *Med Teach* 2012;**34**:205–14.
2 Fish D and Coles C. *Medical Education, Developing a Curriculum for Practice.* Maidenhead: Open University Press, 2005, p. 188.

Chapter 10 **Conclusion**

Assessment is tricky. We know it has to be done but often feel uncomfortable doing it. Assessing was once a mysterious process where judgement was made by experts of their learners without any explanation or justification, against unclear criteria. We then moved to what was perceived to be a fairer and standardised examination of learners conducted in formal settings. Teachers strived to make assessments as objective as possible, applying statistical tests and standard setting measures, which reassured us that the process must be good as 'scientific' numbers were involved. We somehow forgot along the way that judgements by experts were made to get to these numbers. Now assessments within the workplace are evolving further – where we are asked, among other things, to make a global judgement of a learner. In some respects, we have come full circle but now are documenting the process and making it more transparent. Assessment of learners' professionalism is still problematic for a variety of reasons that have been explored in this book.

A note of caution for those who say they have the perfect way of assessing a professional in practice. Coles and Fish describe assessments of learners like X-rays.

> They can only be indicative, and we must not read too much into them, or at least not into one alone. This is because, like x rays, there are no assessment methods that are 100 per cent accurate, every method has false negatives, and any method tells you only about the learners' achievements (patients' condition) at the time, but this will not necessarily predict how they will be in the future. [1]

How to Assess Doctors and Health Professionals, First Edition. Mike Davis, Judy McKimm, and Kirsty Forrest.
© 2013 Blackwell Publishing Ltd. Published 2013 by Blackwell Publishing Ltd.

So, we will leave you with the thought that when thinking about which assessments to use with which learners, the fundamental question to ask is 'What is the purpose of the assessment?' With this in mind, however assessment modalities change in future, you will not go far wrong.

Reference

1 Fish D and Coles C. *Medical Education, Developing a Curriculum for Practice.* Maidenhead: Open University Press, 2005.

Index

Page numbers in *italics* refer to Figures; those in **bold** to Tables.

How to Assess Doctors and Health Professionals, First Edition. Mike Davis, Judy McKimm, and
Kirsty Forrest.
© 2013 Blackwell Publishing Ltd. Published 2013 by Blackwell Publishing Ltd.